SKINFOOD

SKINFOOD

Your 4-Step Solution to
Healthy, Happy Skin

Dr Thivi Maruthappu

PIATKUS

PIATKUS

First published in Great Britain in 2023 by Piatkus

5 7 9 10 8 6 4

A CIP catalogue record for this book
is available from the British Library.

ISBN 978-0-3494-3289-2

Typeset in Sabon by M Rules
Printed and bound in Great Britain by Clays Ltd, Elcograf S.p.A.

Papers used by Piatkus are from well-managed forests
and other responsible sources.

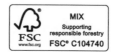

Some names and identifying details have been changed.
This book contains advice and information relating to healthcare.
It should be used to supplement rather than replace the advice of your
doctor or another trained health professional. If you know or suspect
you have a health problem, it is recommended that you seek your
doctor's advice before embarking on any programme or
treatment. All efforts have been made to assure the
accuracy of the information contained in this
book as of the date of publication.

Piatkus
An imprint of Little, Brown Book Group
Carmelite House
50 Victoria Embankment
London EC4Y 0DZ

An Hachette UK Company
www.hachette.co.uk

www.littlebrown.co.uk

In memory of my father, Mahen (1947–2000)
And my granny, Meena (1920–2017)
And for James, Oscar, Rafferty and Atticus
With love

The author will donate 10 per cent of the royalties she receives
from sales of this book in support of skin disease research.

About the Author

Dr Thivi Maruthappu MA PhD FRCP ANutr is a consultant dermatologist, nutritionist and researcher. As the UK's first dual-qualified dermatologist and nutritionist, her pioneering expertise bridges the gap between diet and skin health. Dr Thivi works in the NHS and has her own practice based at London's Cleveland Clinic. She also conducts research on nutrition and the skin at King's College, London, where she is an honorary senior lecturer.

Dr Thivi studied medicine at the University of Oxford and completed her dermatology training in London. She undertook a PhD to investigate the links between our skin and internal health and completed further training in severe eczema and psoriasis at St John's Institute of Dermatology, London, before obtaining a certificate in nutrition science from Stanford Medical School, USA. Over the course of her career, Dr Thivi has garnered numerous academic awards and prizes from organisations including the British Association of Dermatologists, the British Society for Investigative Dermatology and the Royal Society of Medicine.

Dr Thivi lives in north London with her husband and three sons. In her spare time, she loves experimenting with new recipes and roaming Hampstead Heath.

Contents

Introduction:
The 4-Step Skin Solution

Our skin is extraordinary. As our largest organ, it covers the entire surface of our body. Beautifully complex and intelligent, it is also one of the most important ways in which we express ourselves to the outside world. Throughout life, our skin grows, adapts and tells a story. Scars on our knees are a souvenir of childhood accidents, sunspots and freckles remind us of lazy holidays on the beach, and laughter lines form a map of happy memories. Our skin is the tapestry of our life – a culmination of our experiences and who we are.

At this very moment our skin is carrying out an array of important functions, from keeping our temperature in check to protecting us against pollution and harmful ultraviolet rays. Our skin helps us to experience the world around us, with its plethora of nerves allowing us to sense touch, pain and pressure. It has the most remarkable ability to heal, repairing and regenerating itself after scrapes and cuts. Despite its miraculous abilities, our skin is often judged on one simple trait: its appearance.

The world in which we live today has become skin obsessed. We are constantly bombarded with images of flawless, glowing skin everywhere we look, whether that's a billboard, the side of a bus, in magazines or in (often filtered) social-media selfies. The pursuit of clear skin has become the Holy Grail for many.

Throughout history, our skin has represented one of the most important aspects of our identity: at its simplest, it expresses our cultural heritage and race. Although some may be sceptical, there is a longstanding and deeply rooted belief that our skin also reflects our health, well-being and, in some cultures, even social status; for example, in the West, a tan can be seen as a sign of wealth as it signals the ability to afford holidays abroad in the sun, whereas in many Eastern cultures, it's the opposite: fair skin is far more desirable as it suggests wealth and the privilege to remain indoors rather than having to toil in the fields.

Given the emphasis we place on our skin, it's no wonder that we are willing to put so much time, energy and money into achieving a radiant glow. And we've been led to believe that the solution can be found in an assortment of creams and lotions, or, failing that, facials, chemical peels and even more expensive alternatives such as lasers. In short, the skincare industry is booming with eager customers looking for the latest magical skin fix.

What if I told you, however, that the first step in your skincare routine actually starts with what's on your plate? The truth is that what's in your fridge matters just as much as what's in your bathroom, as skincare is both an inside and an outside job. As a consultant dermatologist working in both the NHS and private practice, I have over 15 years of experience with thousands of patients to draw on. My research in nutrition science has led me to combine the latest cutting-edge nutrition advice with skincare and medical treatments to address the most common skin concerns. In this book I'll share my 4-Step Skin Solution to the skin you want that encompasses the 360-degree approach to skin health that I use in my clinic.

Skin and our well-being: my story

How our skin looks and feels has a profound effect on our mood and confidence, so what happens when our skin doesn't live up to our expectations? I have looked after patients with skin conditions of varying levels of severity, from extreme cases of psoriasis to stubborn acne, and one thing that all my patients have in common is a loss of confidence as a result. It is not uncommon for people living with skin conditions to suffer from depression or anxiety. In fact, 98 per cent of people with a skin condition agree that it affects their emotional and psychological well-being.[1] This is all the more reason to treat skin conditions early and effectively.

Your skin can impact every aspect of your life: the relationships you have, the clothes you choose to wear, your job and, of course, your mental health and well-being. I say this not only as a dermatologist, but also as someone who has personal experience of dealing with a skin condition.

Early one summer when I was at university, I developed a painful red rash on my arms after spending the day outdoors in the sun. I didn't think much of it, but the rash slowly grew into painful fluid-filled blisters. Despite trying strong steroid creams from my doctor, the rash wouldn't settle and was so painful and itchy that it was impossible to sleep, and I ended up missing lectures. It persisted for months, worsening every time my skin was exposed to sunlight, and I kept thinking: *how on earth will I cope with this for the rest of my life?*

After seeing several doctors and noticing no improvement, I finally found a dermatologist who was able to diagnose the rash as a rare form of sun sensitivity. I was immediately started on steroid tablets and an immune-suppressing medication called cyclosporine, which changed my skin and my life. I could finally go back to lectures, socialise and enjoy myself. And although everything cleared up fairly quickly, I know that I was very lucky to meet exactly the right doctor who could help.

The experience was a major low point, but it set me on a new career path: I knew I wanted to pursue dermatology, as I understood intimately what it felt like to be trapped by your skin and for it to make you feel completely powerless. I felt so strongly that I wanted to help people in the very same way that I had been helped, and this empathy remains the driving force behind my work. My own experience of a skin condition shows just how profoundly skin can change your life. For me, it shaped my entire career.

Nutrition and the skin

Running a busy dermatology clinic in a large London NHS teaching hospital, I soon became surprised by how many patients asked about nutrition and their skin. From eczema to acne, it was a question that seemed to come up more often than any other.

- Does what I eat affect my skin?
- Should I change my diet to help clear up my skin?
- What about gluten or dairy?

Clearly, it was important to my patients, but why hadn't we learned about it in any dermatology textbooks? Why wasn't it discussed at our regular meetings or conferences? It seemed to me that there was a disconnect between what our patients wanted to know and the information that we were able to provide. I kept coming back to the connection between skin and nutrition, and I wondered why it was easy to explain complex new treatments for conditions such as psoriasis but when asked a simple question about food I was stumped.

I quickly came to the realisation that I was not alone and that my colleagues felt the same. We hadn't received much training in nutrition at medical school, so we didn't feel confident answering questions about it. From all my discussions and conversations with patients, I knew that this wasn't good enough. The problem was that if we weren't able to give answers, patients were resorting to questionable dietary advice found online, attempting extreme fad diets and ending up even more frustrated as a result. We had to do better, and this became my motivation. I then set about reading the extensive research on nutrition and the skin, starting with psoriasis, then moving on to acne, rosacea and eczema. My fascination with the intersection between skin and nutrition evolved quickly into a passion. I realised that it highlighted a void in our knowledge, a blind spot, so to speak, and I became captivated by the potential for nutrition to change the way we cared for the skin.

Eager to find out more, I enrolled myself on a nutrition science course run by the pioneering team at the Stanford School of Medicine. As a busy mum of three boys with a hectic work schedule, I soon discovered that it was no easy feat to add studying to the mix. I found myself waking up at 4am to work on essays and trying to fit in reading and assignments whenever I had a spare moment, but I can safely say that all the hard work was worth it, because understanding nutrition has changed the way I practise. In fact, I now teach fellow dermatologists, nutritionists and dietitians about the connection between nutrition and the skin, and established the nutritional dermatology research group at King's College, London, which is the first of its kind in the UK. Most importantly, I can now offer meaningful answers to my patients' questions about nutrition that are based on science and research.

Four steps to the skin you want

Our skin health is influenced by many different factors in addition to our individual genetics, such as stress, nutrition, sleep and much more. I think of each of these as a piece of a puzzle, and what I have learned from listening to patients over the years is that each piece counts. With that in mind, I've created a 4-Step Skin Solution that will help restore and protect the health of your skin. Here are my four key steps (and don't worry, we'll be doing a deep dive into each a bit later):

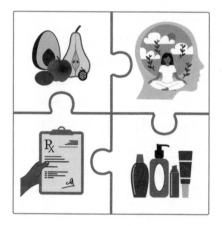

Step 1 Nutrition for skin health
Step 2 The mind–skin connection
Step 3 An effective skincare routine
Step 4 Specialist medical treatments (if required)

During the early years of my career as a dermatologist, I believed that skincare started with a prescription, so I focused on medical treatments as a solution to stubborn skin complaints, prescribing antibiotics to alleviate symptoms of acne or creams to calm eczema. As I started working more with leading skincare brands, I learned the importance of an effective skincare routine and came to appreciate the results that a combination of the right skincare products and prescriptions could deliver. But despite this, I was frustrated. Although I could see visible improvements in my patients' skin, it felt as if there was something missing in my overall approach and that I was treating skin in a, for want of a better word, superficial way.

It was while studying for my PhD that I began to think about skin in a more holistic way, as my research led me to a fascinating connection between internal diseases, such as inherited heart conditions and cancers, and their impact on the skin. By understanding the interplay between skin and health, it became clear to me that the two are intimately connected. I quickly realised that if nutrition acts as the foundation for our overall health, then it also needs to form the first step of any approach to healthy skin.

Developments in the understanding of the mind–body connection have also played a vital role in influencing my philosophy when it comes to treatment. As research increasingly supports, there is an unquestionable relationship between our brain and our skin, which is why the mind–skin connection forms an integral part of my 4-step approach.

By including these two extra steps, I have noticed a profound difference when it comes to my patients' overall skin health. That said, I'm by no means suggesting that skincare isn't fantastic or that medical treatments don't transform lives: of course they do.

But incorporating Step 1 and 2 could be the difference between the results you have and the results you want.

In each section of the 4-Step Skin Solution you'll find tailored advice for the most common concerns I see in the clinic: premature skin ageing/loss of radiance, acne, rosacea, psoriasis and eczema. I have created specific plans around each of these, because the advice I give for someone with rosacea is really quite different from my recommendations for someone with acne. From precision probiotics to guidance around vitamins, I wanted to create an experience that would reflect the bespoke consultation we would have if you came to see me in the clinic. My intention is that this book will show you why skincare is so much more than skin deep. Whether you want to improve the appearance of your skin or find solutions to specific skin issues such as acne, this book will act as your roadmap to healthy skin – something that I truly believe we all deserve.

1

The Fundamentals: Skin School

Our skin is deeply connected to our well-being. Factors such as stress, insomnia, smoking and a diet lacking in nutrients can all dramatically affect how we look. This isn't rocket science, and it's something we've all experienced, me included. As a junior doctor working long, stressful hours, I survived on little sleep, endless coffees and a diet of microwave meals, cafeteria fry-ups and whatever I could get my hands on from the vending machine. Despite taking a handful of vitamins each morning, my skin inevitably suffered, becoming dull and lacklustre. But the good news is that it doesn't have to be that way; making simple changes to your diet and overall sleep hygiene, and lowering your stress levels can yield remarkable results.

In this chapter I'll explain why I consider nutrition and self-care to be the very first steps in any skincare routine, ones you absolutely cannot skip. But before we get there, let's start with the basics and learn more about what makes up our skin and how it functions and what happens when things go awry.

Feeling good in your skin is your birthright, and if you're not quite there yet, don't worry. That's what I'm here for, and we will work slowly and steadily towards happier, healthier skin and renewed confidence through my ground-breaking 4-Step Skin Solution. But before we start implementing any changes to our diet or skincare routine, it's important that we have a solid understanding of the purpose our skin serves and what's really going on underneath the surface. This chapter will teach you all about the skin's make-up, its most important functions, and how and why skin conditions develop, to ensure that you're equipped with the most important information when it comes to your skin. Let's get you enrolled and started in Skin School!

The skin you're in

Our skin is unique to us. From its colour, to the pattern of our moles and birthmarks, it is our irreplaceable blueprint. Identical twins are often studied in medical research due to their matching genetic make-up, but even with the same genes, their skin can differ considerably; for example, one twin might suffer from eczema and the other from acne, and they can even have completely different skin tones. Studying twins helps us to get a better idea of what is caused by nature (our genes) versus nurture (our environment, including diet and stress). It is precisely this variation that makes skin so fascinating. Of course, genetics matters, but what we do, how we live and the way we take care of ourselves plays an important role too.

Despite the many differences between us, the basic structure of the skin varies little from one person to another, independent of our age or ethnicity. Like so many things in life, when we look deeper, we are far more similar than we are different.

The skin is our body's largest organ and responsible for many important functions. It consists of three individual layers that lie on top of one another:

1   The epidermis
2   The dermis
3   The subcutaneous layer

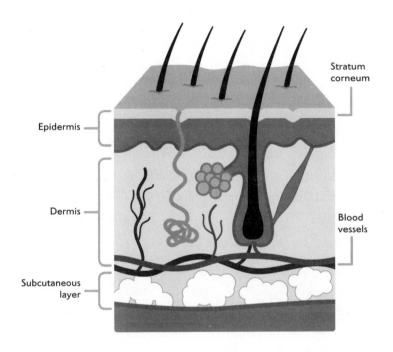

Anatomy of the skin. The skin is made up of three layers:
the epidermis, the dermis and the subcutaneous layer.

Weighing on average 10kg, our skin carries out a multitude of important functions, and, quite clearly, we would not survive without it. In devastating conditions that cause skin failure, such as widespread burns or a severe allergic reaction to medication (known as toxic epidermal necrolysis), the loss of the normal functioning of our skin can even lead to death. I don't mention this to cause alarm but purely to emphasise the point that our skin is not just a covering, it is indispensable for life. The many duties it performs include:

- Regulating body temperature: the skin is our very own thermostat, cooling us down by sweating and keeping us warm by trapping insulating air close to its surface.
- Providing a protective barrier to UV light, chemicals and pollution.
- Acting as a water-resistant barrier.
- Protecting and cushioning us from injury.
- Producing vitamin D and hormones.
- Housing an immune system that fights infection.
- Containing its own microbiome: a collection of beneficial bacteria, yeasts, fungi and viruses that cohabit on the surface of the skin.

Top layer: the epidermis

This is the layer of the skin that we can see. The term epidermis is derived from the Greek word *epi*, meaning outer, and *derma*, which refers to the skin. As you can see from the illustration above, it is the thinnest layer of the skin at around 1mm thick and is made up of four to five layers of skin cells. You've probably noticed that the thickness of your skin varies across the body, and this is largely determined by the epidermis; for example, the epidermis on the soles of our feet is thicker (around 20–30 layers of cells) in order to withstand the pressure of walking, whereas the epidermis around the eyes is very thin (just a single layer) to allow for eye movement and expression. Thin skin around the eyes is particularly susceptible to sun damage and pollution, which is why it often shows the first signs of ageing, such as fine lines and wrinkles.

The epidermis is made up of layers of skin cells called keratinocytes, so called because they contain the protein keratin. Although you may have come across keratin in hair-care products, it functions as a vital protein in the body that gives strength and structure to our hair, skin and nails.

The outermost layer of the epidermis is known as the stratum corneum, which forms our skin barrier. The epidermis is constantly renewing itself, with fresh new cells rising up from the deeper layers, moving to the upper layers where they form a protective barrier.

The process of skin renewal is important in keeping our skin healthy and youthful. In our twenties it takes 28 days for the epidermis to renew, but this process becomes more sluggish as we age and slows to about half this speed by the time we reach our fifties.

The skin barrier

Our skin barrier is our body's first line of defence: it keeps harmful bacteria out and protects us from UV light and pollution. It also retains moisture and prevents the skin from drying out. When our skin barrier isn't working properly, we might notice that our skin becomes dry, flaky and prone to irritation. Over-exfoliating, too much sun and using harsh facial products can all weaken the skin barrier, causing it to become less effective. Skin conditions such as eczema can also develop when the skin barrier is compromised. Think of the skin barrier as a wall made up of a combination of skin cells (bricks) plus fats and fatty compounds known as ceramides (mortar). Amazingly, there are trillions of microorganisms, known collectively as the 'skin microbiome' that also live in the skin. These bugs help to train our immune system and even fight infections on our behalf.

This is my way of saying that our skin barrier is pretty extraordinary. As I explain to my patients, time and time again: look after your skin barrier and it will look after you.

Pigmentation and skin colour

Our individual skin, hair and eye colour are the results of the amounts of melanin pigment we have in the body. In the skin, there are two main types of melanin: eumelanin is responsible for dark colours, such as black and brown, whereas pheomelanin is the type of pigment found in pink areas of skin such as the lips. Both types are produced by skin cells called melanocytes, and although our skin tone can vary, we all have a similar number of melanocytes in the skin. It's how much of each type of melanin our skin makes that dictates the colour of our skin.

The purpose of melanin is to protect us from harmful UV rays and sun damage. When we expose our skin to the sun, it responds by increasing the amount of melanin it makes to darken (or tan) or develop freckles. Lighter skin types don't produce as much eumelanin following sun exposure and therefore tend to burn more easily. It's always important, however, to protect your skin from sunlight with sunscreen and appropriate clothing. This is because UV rays can damage our DNA over time, and repeated burning episodes contribute to both skin cancer and ageing. (I discuss sunscreen and obtaining sufficient levels of vitamin D while using it on page 68.)

Middle layer: the dermis

Below the epidermis sits the thickest layer: the dermis. As you can see from the illustration on page 11, the dermis makes up the bulk of our skin. The dermis is arguably the most important layer when it comes to skin ageing, radiance and glow. Why? I often use the analogy of a sandwich to explain the importance of the dermis. Think of the epidermis and the subcutaneous layers as the bread and the dermis as the filling.

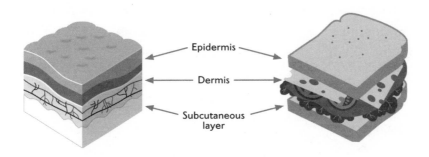

The food we eat nourishes our skin, and the skin's layers can be likened to a sandwich with a nutrient-packed filling: the dermis contains a network of blood vessels that will supply the skin with the nutrients it requires.

We can use the skin/sandwich analogy: the arteries and veins indicate the presence of blood vessels in the dermal layer. Within the dermis this rich network of blood vessels supplies it with essential nutrients required for skin health. Oxygen, vitamins, minerals, proteins and fats are all delivered directly to the skin by blood vessels in the dermis. And where do all these nutrients actually come from, you might ask? The nutrients in the foods we eat are digested and absorbed in the gut and enter our bloodstream, where they are delivered to the skin. From here, nutrients pass from the blood vessels and into the deeper layers of the skin where they support repair and regeneration. This is the first principle of nutrition and skin health: what we eat and drink is digested and delivered to the skin, supplying it with nutrients required for healthy function and specific vitamins that counteract skin ageing.

The dermis also contains nerves that allow us to experience the sensations of touch, pressure, pain and temperature, as well as sweat glands and oil glands that open up to the skin's surface. Sweating helps to regulate our body temperature, and oil (or sebum) keeps the skin moisturised and supple. In short, there's a lot going on in the dermis!

Collagen

Collagen is a protein in the dermis that makes up about 75 per cent of our skin, and you might have noticed that almost all anti-ageing skin treatments, whether creams, injections or even supplements, aim to boost or preserve it. Widely considered the fountain-of-youth protein, collagen provides strength and resilience while also helping skin remain supple. There are twenty-eight different types of collagen in the body, but only types 1 and 3 are found in the skin, so bear this in mind if you're considering taking collagen supplements.

Scientists have made efforts to uncover what makes collagen so unique and have discovered that it's made up of chains of amino acids (the building blocks of all proteins), intertwined to form a rope-like structure. When stretched, these ropes work like a mesh – picture a pair of fishnet tights – that distribute tension evenly before recoiling. Over time, collagen levels naturally drop, which results in the skin losing its bounce and becoming more susceptible to wrinkle formation. This process can be accelerated due to damage caused by pollution, stress and even sugar, but it's UV light that's the number-one culprit. There's a simple way to prove this: compare the skin on your face to a patch of skin that doesn't get much sun, like the inside of your upper arm, and you'll notice that shielded from UV light, this skin retains its youthful appearance for much longer.

Don't worry, though, it's not all doom and gloom! You don't have to give up all sugar and beach holidays forever, as we can naturally look after and maintain our collagen levels with sensible sun protection and by making changes to our diet, and this is something we'll cover in more detail when I introduce you to the SkinFood Approach in Chapter 4.

Fibroblasts

Within the dermis lie fibroblasts, cellular powerhouses that produce collagen, and the hydrating molecule, hyaluronic acid, among other proteins. Like all skin cells, fibroblasts are vulnerable to UV damage, and over time they become depleted and sluggish, with our skin suffering as a result.

Fibroblasts also play a critical role in wound healing; for example, when we scrape our knee, they multiply and produce essential chemical messengers to promote healing, stimulating the production of collagen, elastin and other growth factors. This is also why you might notice that your cuts take longer to heal as you get older. As we age, our skin requires more time to recover. Babies and small children have the highest numbers of fibroblasts in their skin, which results in smooth, plump skin that heals remarkably well.

Fibroblasts are heavily dependent on specific nutrients to do their job; these include carbohydrates, proteins and fats, as well as micronutrients such as vitamins C, D and E, zinc, iron, selenium and copper. This is the reason why a nutrient-dense diet is important for proper wound healing; for example, with scarring from skin conditions such as acne.

Bottom layer: the subcutaneous tissue

The subcutaneous layer describes the cushion of fat and connective tissue that lies between the dermis and underlying muscles. It will vary depending on its location in the body; you might see, for example, on the back of your hands that there is very little fat padding, but at other sites, such as the stomach, the layers are much thicker.

A plump face has long been associated with a youthful appearance, so losing subcutaneous fat, particularly around your face, can be ageing. Think of fat as our natural filler that needs to be supported through diet, so try to work in plenty of good fats from nuts, seeds and healthy oils into your daily meals (more on how to do this in Chapter 4).

Making the connection – why nutrition matters

In recent years, a growing body of scientific research has shown how important a role nutrition plays when tackling a whole range of skin concerns. As I mentioned earlier, it's also become a cornerstone of my own clinical research and practice, and this is because paying attention to nutrition can be transformative.

While there are universal nutritional principles that should be adopted no matter what your skin type, there are also specific dietary suggestions that take into account individual skin concerns.

How does the food we eat actually affect our skin?

Starting with the fundamental principles, our skin needs nutrients, a balance of protein, carbohydrates and fats as well as vitamins and minerals, to function properly and support renewal and repair. Skin cells are no different from any other cells in our body in this respect, but our skin, hair and nails are some of the first places that show signs of a nutrient deficiency. Low levels of essential good fats such as omega-3 will contribute to dehydrated, flaky skin and dry, dull hair. In the next chapter, we'll look in greater detail at how low levels of particular nutrients can cause skin symptoms and how these can be remedied through diet or the right supplements.

Beyond this, specific foods and the nutrients they contain can have other consequences on the skin. These can broadly be categorised into 'direct' and 'indirect' responses. Sometimes the relationship between what we eat and what happens to our skin is simply a matter of cause and effect, as is the case with food allergies; that is, if we eat something that we are allergic to, we can expect a reaction in the form of blotching or wheals.

CASE STUDY: A CURIOUS RASH

I remember some years ago, a young man came to the clinic as an emergency patient. He had come out in a rash with bright red wheals all over his back that looked like scratch marks. Curious, I asked if he had been scratching his back, but he assured me that he hadn't and that the marks had suddenly appeared out of nowhere. The rash was distinctive, and although I recognised it from my medical textbooks, I'd never seen it in person before. The next step was to ask the patient what he'd recently eaten, and specifically whether he'd had any mushrooms. It turned out he had drunk shiitake tea at a health-food store the day before so I deduced that the rash was an incredibly rare case of shiitake mushroom dermatosis.[1]

As a dermatologist you're likely to see the rash described above only once in a lifetime, if at all. It's triggered by a reaction to a component in undercooked shiitake mushrooms called lentinan. In some cases, lentinan will react with cells in the body to cause skin inflammation. The rash in this young man was a perfect example. Although exciting for me, it was not so exciting for the patient. Luckily for him, however, the rash settled quickly and all he had to do was avoid undercooked shiitake mushrooms in the future. This is a clear example of how joining the dots between what we eat and our skin can sometimes be straightforward and occasionally surprising.

The most familiar direct reaction between food and skin is an allergy: eat something you are sensitive to and you'll come out in hives: your skin will be itchy and you might start developing swelling pretty quickly. The reaction that foods such as nuts or shellfish can trigger in at-risk individuals sets off a cascade of histamine release, causing redness and wheals on the skin that can even lead to life-threatening anaphylaxis.

For others, certain foods can have an indirect effect by precipitating flare-ups of a skin condition. Rosacea, for example, can be worsened by spicy foods and alcohol. This type of reaction isn't a food allergy, but it is caused instead by the sensitivity of blood vessels in the face to those foods and drinks.

Food and the nutrients that it contains can have other indirect effects on the skin. What we consume can influence our hormones, such as insulin; for example, a diet high in refined sugar from sweets and biscuits causes raised blood sugar and insulin levels, which in some people can trigger acne and breakouts. What and when we eat also influences our gut health, which refers to the trillions of organisms that reside in our gut. Scientific advances over the last decade have shone a light on the exciting relationship between gut health and the skin, and we'll look more closely at this vital link in Chapter 3.

What your skin is trying to tell you

As the interface between our external and internal worlds, the skin acts as a window into our health, and changes in its appearance can provide clues to our overall well-being. This is a powerful principle that allows medical professionals to identify a myriad of conditions, such as type-2 diabetes and even heart disease, years before other symptoms occur, just by carrying out a little detective work and studying a patient's skin. Here is an easy example of this idea in action: pinch the skin on the back of your hands and look at whether it recoils immediately. If you're severely dehydrated, your skin won't snap back and will wrinkle instead regardless of age. But this idea extends beyond just the skin: both the hair and nails are also useful indicators of what's really going on in your body. Changes in our nails can indicate anaemia, liver disease or even a hidden cancer. The face holds many signs too, as yellowish spots around the eyes can indicate high cholesterol, which is one of the most important risk factors for heart attacks and strokes, whereas the colour of your inner eyelids can go some way to indicating whether you might have anaemia.

For me, understanding the way our skin reflects our internal health has been one of the most fascinating aspects of dermatology, and it is what I chose to focus on when studying for my PhD at Queen Mary University of London, supervised by leading experts Professor David Kelsell and Professor Edel O'Toole. My research involved investigating rare skin conditions and learning what they could teach us about our health. One particular study still stands out to me. I was exploring a heart condition called arrhythmogenic cardiomyopathy (ACM), which can cause sudden cardiac arrest and death, and as part of this research I met families who had lost loved ones to ACM. I spoke to them, examined their skin and hair, and looked at photos of their lost relatives. The affected family members were all found to carry a faulty gene responsible for the heart condition, and this fault meant that they were at a much higher risk of developing the disease. The gene in question is responsible for making a protein called desmoplakin, which is supposed to glue heart cells together. The genetic mutation meant that the desmoplakin couldn't function properly and it was no longer an effective glue. As a result, electrical signals misfired, resulting in an irregular heartbeat. Over time, the irregular electrical heartbeats can go haywire and prove deadly.

What does this have to do with skin? Strikingly, we observed that the majority of affected family members who carried the faulty gene had a few things in common: tightly curled, 'wire-wool' hair and a rare skin condition affecting their feet called keratoderma. In fact, I could often spot the patients who carried the mutations as they sat in the waiting room just by looking out for their tightly curled hair.

We soon realised that the very same protein that was faulty in the heart was also faulty in the skin and hair. As desmoplakin also glues skin cells together, weak connections between skin and hair cells were causing the curly, frizzy hair and keratoderma that we noticed in patients. Essentially, what is happening in the heart is perfectly mirrored in the skin. This ground-breaking discovery connecting the skin and the heart made waves, and our research was published in the *British Journal of Dermatology*[2] and featured widely in the press. This new knowledge will be used to identify people at high risk of developing a deadly heart condition, and clues found in the skin and hair will save lives.

In the table below I have listed just a few examples of skin rashes and how they can be linked to other medical conditions. This list isn't meant to help you self-diagnose but merely to illustrate how intricately our skin health and overall health are intertwined. It goes without saying that clear skin does not mean you are free from all illness, while having a rash doesn't mean that you are suffering from an internal disease, either.

Skin rash (medical name)	Appearance	Linked medical conditions
Jaundice	Yellowish discolouration of the skin and eyes	Liver disease
Dermatitis herpetiformis	Itchy bumps and blisters on elbows and knees	Coeliac disease (auto-immune reaction to gluten in wheat)
Vitiligo	Patches/areas of skin with a loss of pigmentation	Thyroid disease, type-1 diabetes, anaemia caused by low levels of B12
Pruritus	Itchy skin	Anaemia caused by low iron
Acanthosis nigricans	Thickened velvety, darkened skin in the armpits, neck and groin	Hormonal imbalances such as polycystic ovaries and type-2 diabetes. Can rarely be linked to some cancers

Skin rashes and their link to other medical conditions.

For too long the skin has been seen as simply an external barrier, almost entirely separate from the rest of our body, but it's so much more than that. Our skin is inextricably linked with our overall health, which is why taking steps towards improving nutrition and lifestyle habits can make all the difference to the appearance of our skin.

Common skin concerns and their causes

Now that we have a better understanding of the make-up of our skin and its many functions, it's time to turn our attention to appreciating why specific skin concerns arise and how we might go about treating them.

NOTE This isn't an exhaustive list of skin conditions by any means, but these are the most common complaints that I see in the clinic: acne, premature skin ageing or loss of radiance, rosacea, eczema and psoriasis.

Acne

Acne is the single most common skin concern that I see in the clinic, and it's fair to say that almost all of us have experienced spots, zits, pimples or breakouts at some time or another. Fortunately, it's also very treatable, and I like to use the 4-Step Skin Solution with my patients to ensure that we're treating the symptoms of acne and the causes. Acne is not simply a skin condition: it can have a profound impact on how we feel about ourselves, our confidence and self-esteem, so it's important to treat it in a holistic way.

Why does acne happen?

First, let's look at what really causes acne and debunk some enduring myths with the following table:

Myth	Fact
Acne only affects teens	Acne often first appears during the teenage years due to hormonal fluctuations, but it can persist into adulthood or present for the first time at any age, including around the menopause
Acne is caused by a 'bad diet'	For some people, certain foods can trigger acne flare-ups; however, this is not the cause of acne. It is most often caused by a combination of genetics and hormonal factors
Sunbeds clear up acne	You might notice that acne clears up in the summer months, but sunbeds are not the answer, as they increase the risk of skin cancer and premature ageing in the longer term
Squeezing spots will get rid of acne more quickly	Squeezing spots can increase the risk of permanent scars and can spread bacteria
You can catch acne from someone else	Acne is not contagious!

The myths and facts about acne.

It might surprise you to learn that the majority of acne patients I see in my clinic are adults. It's a very common misconception that acne only affects teens, when in fact about 40 per cent of adult men and almost half of all adult women experience breakouts too.

What does acne look like?

Acne is an inflammatory condition that affects a part of the skin known as the pilosebaceous unit, which is essentially a hair follicle attached to a sebaceous (oil) gland. It most commonly affects the face, chest and back. The hair itself may or may not be visible, but our pores form the opening of the follicles. As you can see in the illustration below, there are four steps in the forming of a pimple.

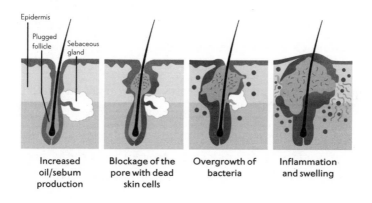

| Increased oil/sebum production | Blockage of the pore with dead skin cells | Overgrowth of bacteria | Inflammation and swelling |

The timeline of a pimple.

We used to think that acne was caused by a skin infection, but we now understand that it is the combination of blockage, inflammation and bacteria on the surface of the skin that gives rise to skin breakouts. The term 'acne' or 'pimple' describes many different types of skin lesion. This explains why acne can look very different on different parts of your face and body, and it can vary from person to person.

Closed comedone A pore clogged with oil, dead skin and bacteria can result in a raised, flesh-coloured bump on the surface of the skin. These are also known as whiteheads due to the waxy whitish substance, which you can just see under the surface of the skin.

Open comedone A clogged pore may remain flesh coloured, but following exposure to the air, oxidisation can occur and the colour of the contents changes from white/yellow to dark brown/black. This is known as a blackhead. It is tempting to try to squeeze blackheads, but you risk scarring your skin in the process. There are more effective ways of managing them with skincare, such as applying retinoids.

Inflammatory papules and pustules Red, warm and tender spots can develop when bacteria within the pore overgrow and this triggers inflammation. The pressure that builds up within the pore can lead to it becoming sore. Depending on the extent of the inflammation, this can be very painful. In some cases, inflammation progresses and your immune system sends white blood cells into the follicle, which causes pus to build up. This rises to the tip of the bump and results in a pustule, which you may be able to see on the surface of the skin. Again, it can be tempting to squeeze these, but proceed with caution, as you might inadvertently drive inflammation deeper in the skin and leave scarring.

Cysts and nodules Nodules are deeper and more painful solid acne lesions that lie in the dermis, the deeper layer of the skin. Because they are located in the dermis, inflammation can disrupt the collagen and elastin fibres that are present here. Consequently, nodules and cysts are much more likely to cause scarring such as pitting. Cysts differ from nodules, as they are pus-filled and inflamed, but as they are located in the deep layers of the skin, trying to squeeze them can be painful and there is a high likelihood of scarring.

What really causes acne?

Like so many skin conditions, acne is the result of many different factors, but it's our individual genetics and hormones that are likely to lay the foundation for oily, acne-prone skin. However, for some, dietary triggers, stress and skincare products or make-up can also have an effect. Genetics explain why some people never get spots, irrespective of their hormones, how much sugar they eat or how much stress they are under. Although acne is driven by genes and hormones, by identifying and addressing individual triggers, such as stress or certain foods, you can learn to work with your skin rather than against it.

To help identify your potential acne triggers so that we can tackle them together, I've summarised the questions that I usually ask when seeing a patient in the clinic:

Potential trigger	Question
Genetics	How long have you had acne? Does anyone in your family have acne?
Hormones	Did your acne flare during your teens/puberty? Does it flare before or around your period? Did it start during the perimenopausal period? Has your acne appeared since starting a hormonal treatment (pill/implant/coil/HRT)? Does your acne commonly occur along the cheeks and jawline?

Polycystic ovarian syndrome (PCOS)	Are your periods irregular or absent at times? Have you noticed hair loss on the scalp? Have you noticed excess unwanted hair growth in areas such as the chin or nipples? Does your acne often occur on the cheeks/ jawline?
Stress	Are you under more stress than usual? Does this cause breakouts to flare? Are you sleeping poorly or working long hours?
Nutrition	Are you taking any vitamin supplements or protein powders? Does your acne flare up after eating certain foods; for example milk, sugary foods? What is your overall diet like?
Skincare and make-up	Are you using pore-blocking products (comedogenic) containing oils? Do you cleanse effectively twice a day? Do you remove make-up before exercising?

Potential triggers for acne.

Hormones and acne

Acne can first appear at times of hormonal fluctuations, most commonly during puberty. In addition, hormonal changes around pregnancy and perimenopause can also cause breakouts in women.

Adolescent acne Acne affects almost 95 per cent of teens. In the past, adolescent acne was often considered less of a priority for treatment, as it was seen as just a phase that teenagers would ultimately grow out of; however, now we have a much better understanding that treating acne at any age matters, as it can seriously impact self-confidence and contribute to scarring that is more difficult to treat later in life. I encourage my patients to adopt steps 1–3 of the 4-Step Skin Solution to soothe teenage acne, which in practice means maintaining a balanced nutritious diet, managing stress where possible and creating an effective skincare routine. For many this will keep breakouts at bay, but Step 4 can also be introduced, if needed.

Pre-menstrual acne Pre-menstrual flare-ups of acne are incredibly common. I'm sure you won't be surprised to learn that over half of all women with acne notice pesky spots surfacing just before their monthly period. This is because levels of the hormones oestrogen and progesterone drop in advance of menstruation, while levels of androgens (such as testosterone) remain constant throughout the month, and as a result they become relatively higher in comparison. We know that androgens drive sebum production in the skin and can provoke breakouts, and for many women these flare-ups will occur around the jawline and chin area. Studies have examined whether women with hormonal acne have abnormal levels of hormones, but this does not consistently seem to be the case. Instead, it's believed that those who suffer with hormonal acne have skin that is more sensitive to the hormones. Keeping blood sugar steady can also help hormonal fluctuations and we will look at how to do this in Chapter 4.

Perimenopausal acne It may be surprising to know that acne can also flare up during the perimenopausal period, which includes before, during and sometimes even after the menopause. In this phase, levels of oestrogen start to drop and you may notice that your periods become lighter with longer gaps between them. Like other types of adult female acne, breakouts tend to favour the jawline and chin area. In the same way as we see with premenstrual flares, falling oestrogen levels lead to relatively higher levels of androgens that encourage acne. If you're experiencing perimenopausal acne there are many ways to clear it, including the right skincare and hormonal treatments.

Male acne Male adult acne is more common than you'd think. It is usually a result of genetics and fluctuations in the male hormone testosterone, which drives sebum production, resulting in the skin becoming congested and pimples forming. Some men can experience very severe forms of acne and this is believed to be down to the effects of testosterone. Additionally, the beard area can be a trap for bacteria that contributes to acne development affecting the cheeks and chin. Males are also more commonly prone to back acne, made worse by the accumulation of sweat during workouts. Using a medicated body wash after exercise can be helpful in clearing 'bacne' and we cover ingredients and options in Step 3.

Breakouts caused by whey protein powder tend to occur more frequently in males too, but switching to plant-based protein powders or getting protein from food sources instead can help. Anabolic steroids and testosterone supplements used to increase muscle mass should also be avoided as they are strongly linked to acne.

Acne in skin of colour

Acne can affect people of any skin tone, but there are some important differences to consider in people with darker skin.[3] In deeper skin tones acne can leave persistent dark marks on the skin, known as post-inflammatory pigmentation, and these marks can take months or in some cases even longer to fade and can be an immense source of distress. When treating acne in people with darker skin tones, early and effective treatment must be prioritised to prevent such pigmentation from developing. I recommend treating acne with ingredients that work for both inflammation and pigmentation simultaneously. When choosing products, look for azelaic acid and retinoids in the ingredient list. Combine these with a non-comedogenic (non-pore blocking) SPF to help tackle pigmentation before it has a chance to develop. You'll find much more on skincare for acne in Step 3.

When to seek help with acne

Although there is a lot that you can do to help ameliorate your acne at home, in certain instances I would suggest speaking with a doctor. This is my list of acne red flags:

- If it is affecting your mental health, such as causing a loss of confidence or low self-worth, anxiety or depression.
- If you have painful cysts or nodules (lumps under the skin).
- If acne is resulting in scarring or pigmentation that does not fade.
- If your acne is linked to scalp hair loss, irregular periods or extra hair growth on the face or body.

- If breakouts are not responding to over-the-counter treatments.

How do you treat acne?

Many people with acne turn to their skincare routine as a first course of action in improving their skin health, but this is not my approach. Although products can go a long way to support healthy skin, think back to the pillars of the 4-Step Skin Solution. When tackling acne in the clinic I start with Steps 1–3, as they lay the foundation for healthy skin by promoting a nutritious diet, managing stress levels, focusing on quality sleep and putting an effective skincare routine in place. I will then recommend targeted medical treatments (Step 4) to address stubborn breakouts, if needed. As you read through the book you will be able to understand in detail how these steps work in synchrony to benefit you and your skin.

Premature ageing and the desire for radiant skin

The mission to try to turn back the clock with anti-ageing products has evolved into a multi-billion-pound industry, driven by a myriad of creams and injectable treatments or more drastic surgical procedures. Although the skin over our entire body matures over time, it is the changes to our face that often elicit the most concern. Rather than fighting to reverse ageing, my approach is to preserve and protect our skin from the inside and out. Our skin can be radiant and healthy at any age, if we know how to look after it.

Ageing well is an inside job

So much of the beauty industry is concerned with the visible changes of skin ageing. By focusing solely on the exterior and looking for quick fixes to remain youthful, we are forgetting that ageing well is an inside job. We can preserve our appearance for as long as possible by following a nutritious diet and taking care of our health, but eventually the ageing process itself will win. In addition to how we look, we want to feel good, vibrant and healthy, and we can do this at any age.

My grandmother is one of my greatest inspirations. She died aged 96 without ever having required any medications. She ate well, walked for over an hour daily, meditated for 1 hour three times per day and kept her brain sharp. She would ring each member of her extended family on their birthday, remembering the date and their telephone number without any written prompt. She was truly an inspiration in every way.

She had a beauty that radiated from within. She nourished her mind, body and soul, and although she was richly covered in wrinkles, she was entirely fulfilled. I would love to change the narrative around ageing and focus on ageing well rather than 'anti-ageing', which has far too negative a connotation for my liking. We all want to look our best for as long as possible, and I am certainly no exception, but accepting that we will age and that we won't look the same forever is best for both our physical and mental health.

How does the skin age and why?

The question of how and why we age has captured the imagination of researchers across the globe. We broadly divide skin ageing into two categories: intrinsic and extrinsic. Intrinsic ageing is determined by our genes and is sometimes referred to as 'chronological ageing'. Simply put, it is ageing due to the passage of time, and this isn't something that we can alter. This is a biological process that occurs naturally in all living creatures.

By contrast, extrinsic ageing is within our control and the 4-Step Skin Solution effectively tackles the major components of extrinsic ageing so that you look and feel your best.

Are we actually as young as we look?

Researchers from Denmark have found that how old you look may actually reflect how well you're ageing on the inside. In the largest twin study of its kind published in the *British Medical Journal,*[4] scientists set about estimating the age of twins based on facial photographs. What they found was astonishing, namely that the younger-looking twin lived longer than their older-looking sibling. They concluded that perceived age – how old you look – was a robust biomarker of ageing. It seems as though we are as young as we look.

The researchers were also able to discover that looking younger correlated with having longer telomeres. Telomeres are the caps that sit at the ends of strands of DNA, often likened to the tip at the end of a shoelace that stops it from unravelling. Telomere length determines how often a cell can replicate and renew, and shorter telomeres indicate faster ageing and are linked to many diseases. Unsurprisingly, telomere shortening is accelerated by lifestyle choices such as a poor diet, lack of exercise and smoking, and all these also speed up the ageing process in the skin. This study, along with many others points to the important role that a healthy lifestyle plays in skin ageing.

In women, hormonal changes linked to the menopause are an additional factor that contributes to intrinsic ageing. Falling oestrogen levels lead to reduced collagen production in the dermis; this accelerates the appearance of fine lines and wrinkles. We can make important adjustments to our diet to help counteract fluctuating oestrogen levels associated with the perimenopause and menopause.

Essentially, extrinsic ageing is the sum of all the things that our skin is exposed to over the course of a lifetime. Each one impacts how well our skin ages and how radiant and healthy it looks. Collectively, we refer to these external forces as the 'exposome': nutrition, smoking, alcohol, sun exposure, sleep quality, stress and pollution.[5] How we age is the summation of our intrinsic age (our genes) and the exposome. The 4-Step Skin Solution moves beyond just skincare to address each facet of the exposome so that our skin health is protected and preserved for the future.

UV light and free radicals UV light has long been established as one of the most important factors for skin ageing. Too much time in the sun results in uneven skin tone, fine lines and loss of skin elasticity, and this is often referred to as 'photoageing'. UV also triggers damage to DNA that contributes to the formation of skin cancer.

Although UV light impacts all three layers of the skin, it's the skin's deepest layer, the dermis, that is most severely affected by exposure. Damage to the dermis can have a knock-on effect on the overall appearance of the skin, as it's where collagen can be found. Collagen is arguably the most important protein when it comes to achieving that smooth healthy glow that we're all looking for, so it's essential that we protect it.

Sunlight stimulates the formation of free radicals, which are unstable molecules that try to grab electrons from other molecules. They are produced not only following sun exposure but also by normal metabolic processes in the body. Free radicals attack our DNA and trigger enzymes called matrix metalloproteinases, which break down collagen and elastin. This results in the epidermis growing thicker, the dermis thinner with thin, poorly formed collagen fibres and the subcutaneous fat becoming diminished. These structural changes in the skin contribute to the visible signs of skin ageing and the loss of radiance that we are all familiar with as we age.

What can we do to protect our skin? Fortunately, there are many ways that we can protect our skin from the harmful effects of free radicals, through our diet and skincare. Not only can these tools help to dampen the effects of accelerated ageing in the skin, but they also improve glow.

I am sure you're aware how obsessed dermatologists and skin specialists are with sunscreen: we recommend its use every day because UV light is a major component of skin ageing. But while sunscreen is essential, it isn't the only way we can fight free-radical damage. Within the skin are powerful compounds called antioxidants that can neutralise the effect of free radicals produced by UV light before they are able to cause harm. There are many potent antioxidants in the human body, and several are in the form of vitamins such as vitamin C, E and B, so by ensuring that we have adequate amounts of each through our diet, we can help to mitigate the effects of free radicals on our skin.

Brightly coloured fruits and vegetables are the cornerstone of a skin-friendly diet. Berries are known to contain the highest levels of potent antioxidants, which is also the secret to their rich colour, as their natural antioxidants protect them from UV light. In fact, there are thousands of antioxidant compounds found in fruit and vegetables, which is why it's so important to include as many as possible in your diet.

Most people try to boost radiance and address premature skin ageing by focusing on skincare (Step 3) and occasionally through medical treatments like facial peels, botox and laser therapy. My advice is to also focus on what's on your plate and to consider the mind–skin connection, and your skin will start to thank you.

Rosacea

Rosacea is a common skin condition that causes the face to flush. It affects about 10 per cent of the population, more commonly women, and particularly those who have fair skin or have been exposed to the sun for prolonged periods of time. Blushing is a common feature of rosacea.

As well as visible redness, rosacea can lead to an uncomfortable stinging or burning sensation in the skin and can trigger break-outs. It can also lead to more sensitive skin, which is thought to be a result of the skin barrier not working quite as it should and causing dryness and irritation. One of the characteristics of rosacea is that it can flare up in response to certain triggers:

- UV light
- Temperature changes
- Alcohol
- Spicy foods
- Hot drinks
- Stress

What initially causes rosacea?

We don't fully understand why rosacea occurs, but it seems to result from a combination of genetics, inflammation, reactive blood vessels in the skin and hormonal factors. Blood vessels sitting close to the surface of the skin lead to the appearance of redness, and these vessels are hyper-sensitive to certain triggers. This causes them to widen and results in flushing. Skin inflammation is another feature of rosacea and this can lead to spots and swelling. Initially, redness comes and goes, but with time it can become more persistent.

As you can see from the above list of rosacea triggers, certain foods can aggravate the condition. It is thought that this is the result of blood vessels and nerves in the face being more sensitive to ingredients contained within certain foods, such as anything spicy. In Chapter 5, we will learn more about triggers, and explore how to work out your personal triggers and how to avoid them.

The skin microbiome can also play a role in rosacea and drive inflammation. One organism in particular, a tiny mite called demodex, is found in higher numbers on the skin of people who have the more spot-prone type of rosacea, known as papulopustular rosacea.[6] Fortunately, there are excellent ways to target this mite with prescription skincare (Step 4).

Through research a very important link between rosacea and

the gut microbiome – the trillions of beneficial bacteria that are housed in our digestive system – has been discovered. This has provided new insights into rosacea and a phenomenon called 'the gut–skin link' (we'll do a deep dive into this fascinating area in Chapter 3, but for now back to rosacea).

How do I know if I have rosacea?

The typical symptoms and signs of rosacea are:

- Redness or enlarged blood vessels affecting the centre of the face.
- Red spots in a similar area.
- Blushing or flushing of the face; for example, in response to heat or certain foods.
- The skin feels sensitive, tight and reacts to new skincare products.
- Eye problems, such as dry/gritty eyes can also occur.

It is very easy to confuse rosacea with other common skin conditions such as eczema or acne, as the symptoms and appearance can overlap. It is extremely important to make sure you know which skin condition you have, however, because treatments for eczema and acne can make rosacea substantially worse. If you have any doubt, your doctor or dermatologist should be able to help you.

Although rosacea is often considered a skin condition of lighter skin tones, it can also occur in skin of colour. As redness may not be obvious in skin of colour, it can often be overlooked or misdiagnosed. It helps to pay attention to how skin feels – tightness and stinging, for example – as well as how it looks.

There are four broad types of rosacea and the treatment for

each might differ, but it's worth bearing in mind that it's possible to have more than one type. Here is a brief breakdown of each type:

1 For some people, rosacea presents as redness and flushing in the centre of the face. There may also be prominent red blood vessels visible on the cheeks or nose. Skin can be dry and sensitive, and can sting or burn when skincare products are applied. This is known as erythematotelangiectatic rosacea or ET Rosacea.

2 For others, rosacea can resemble acne with pustules and red lumps (papules) in the central areas of the face. Facial swelling and dry eyes can also develop. This is known as papulopustular rosacea.

3 In more advanced rosacea, the skin of the nose can become thickened, swollen and red – this is much more common in men than women.

4 Rosacea can also affect the eyes and eyelids with symptoms such as gritty dry eyes, burning or stinging. This is known as ocular rosacea and can be treated with warm eye compresses and moisturising eye drops.

How do you treat rosacea?

The causes of rosacea are diverse, and there are many different influences that drive flare-ups, so effective treatment often takes a multi-pronged approach to ensure that each cause is targeted simultaneously. Although this may sound complicated, in the following chapters I'll break down how this can be done using the 4-Step Skin Solution.

Psoriasis

The inflammatory skin condition, psoriasis, is characterised by red scaly patches on the body, which can be itchy and sore. It tends to occur most commonly in adults, and one million people in the UK experience some form of the condition. Much of my training and research has revolved around psoriasis, which I find both fascinating and immensely rewarding to treat. In the last decade, our understanding of why psoriasis happens and how to treat it has made major advancements, and I've incorporated these findings into my tailored approach to treatment.

Why does psoriasis happen?

It is believed that psoriasis arises as the culmination of our individual genes and their impact on the immune system. In psoriasis, an overactive immune system speeds up skin cell growth and turnover, which results in redness, inflammation and scaling.

Environmental triggers can also play a role in affecting when and why psoriasis flares occur. Although we don't fully understand all the environmental triggers responsible, these are thought to be the key ones:

Stress
Trauma to the skin
Infection
Alcohol/smoking
Obesity and nutrition
Hormonal changes
Certain medications

What does psoriasis look like?

Plaque psoriasis is the most common type and is seen in around 80 per cent of people with the condition. It typically appears as round, pink-red raised patches of skin with white scales over the surface. It favours certain areas of the body such as the scalp, belly button, elbows and knees. There are also other types of psoriasis, which can look different:

Guttate psoriasis These are small raindrop-like patches of psoriasis that can spread quite quickly over the body. The trigger is often a throat infection caused by the *Streptococcus* bacterium.

Flexural psoriasis occurs in body creases such as the armpits, groin and behind the ears.

Nail psoriasis Changes in the appearance of the nails, with thickening or small indents, are a common feature of psoriasis.

Pustular psoriasis This type of psoriasis is characterised by pus-filled white spots on red scaly skin. This type can also be limited to just the hands and feet (known as palmoplantar pustular psoriasis).

Psoriasis can look quite different depending on skin tone, with patches more likely to appear dusky rather than red in skin of colour. Psoriasis can also be linked to a type of inflammation in the joints called psoriatic arthritis, and this typically affects around a third of people with psoriasis. Signs include stiffness, swelling and pain in the joints. If you think you might have any of these symptoms, it's important to see your doctor as soon as possible, as this is a condition that benefits from early treatment.

In my experience, the amount of psoriasis you have doesn't always correlate with how much it has an impact on you. Having psoriasis on visible body sites such as the face and hands can be just as distressing (if not more) than having it all over the body in covered locations. Psoriasis can impact your relationships with others, your emotional well-being and stress levels too. We look at ways to address this in Chapter 7.

Can we treat psoriasis?

For several years I led a large psoriasis clinic in a densely populated area of London. Many of my patients came from ethnic minorities and low-income households. I learned more from these patients than in any other role. And although we cannot cure psoriasis, we are generally able to help patients achieve their goal of clearer skin so that they can go back to living their lives.

I am acutely aware that psoriasis is so much more than just a skin condition and that it is connected to our overall health and well-being. Nutrition is now a pivotal part of how I manage psoriasis and linked conditions in the clinic. Addressing important aspects of health alongside skincare and medical treatments, if needed, is a recipe that delivers impact.

Eczema

Dry, itchy and flaky skin, poor sleep and sore, painful patches: if you live with eczema or know someone who does, these symptoms are likely to be very familiar to you. Eczema is a common skin condition, affecting one in five children and one in ten adults in the UK. There are several types of eczema (discoid, pompholyx and contact eczema, to name but a few), but in this book we will primarily focus on atopic eczema, which causes an itchy rash and is often linked to other allergic conditions such as asthma and hayfever.

Eczema can affect any age group, but it often first appears in childhood. Many children outgrow their eczema as they enter their teens, but it can persist or even reappear in adulthood. You might be surprised to learn that it's also possible to develop eczema for the first time as an adult.

Why does eczema happen?

Eczema is by and large influenced by our genes and often runs in families, so if you have eczema, it's likely that members of your family also suffer from it or have a related condition such as asthma or hayfever.

The major gene responsible for eczema is called filaggrin, and up to 50 per cent of people with eczema will have a fault in this gene.[7] Filaggrin is essential for maintaining the integrity of our skin barrier, and it does this by flattening and bundling the outermost layer of skin cells together to create a strong and resilient wall of cells. When filaggrin doesn't work properly, the bricks (cells) in the wall (barrier) don't line up properly and the barrier is weakened, causing the skin to lose moisture and dry out. This is particularly problematic for people with eczema, as they already produce fewer natural oils in the skin.

A weakened skin barrier also allows microbes and allergens in the environment such as dust to irritate the skin. The immune system in people with eczema is often overzealous and reacts to harmless microbes and allergens on the skin, which leads to further irritation and inflammation.

What does eczema look like?

Eczema can differ from person to person, and its appearance is influenced by age, skin tone and the type of eczema. Most commonly, dry itchy patches are present on the elbow creases and behind the knees. In some cases, eczema can become widespread and affect much of the skin.

What does eczema feel like?

The itching associated with eczema is one of the main reasons people come to see me, as it can interfere with sleep, work and well-being. Eczema can also leave the skin feeling dry, tight and uncomfortable – and it can be extremely painful. Living with the condition can take a toll on our mental well-being, and this is something that I'm acutely aware of. I'll offer guidance on how to use proven, science-backed techniques to help you cope (see Chapter 9).

Does food cause eczema?

The unpredictability of eczema is a real challenge: some days things can be quiet, and on other days it can flare up and be hard to pinpoint the triggers. Many people with eczema worry about food: they have concerns about allergies and intolerances, but there can be a lot of confusion surrounding these two separate types of reaction. I'll go through this in detail in Chapter 6 and explain how you can work out if food is playing a role in your eczema. Although food is unlikely to be the cause of eczema, food *allergies* can make eczema worse. We now also understand that the gut microbiome can influence eczema, and we will explore this fascinating research and what it means for you in Chapter 3.

How do you treat eczema, and can you cure it?

Although we do not have a cure for eczema yet, the 4-Step Skin Solution will help to get it under control, and we'll explore how to do this over the course of this book.

Key skin-friendly takeaways

Understanding the anatomy of our skin explains just why it is so incredibly sensitive to changes in our body, including our nutrition and stress levels. This is also why our skin can be seen as a window into our overall health, offering clues to otherwise hidden conditions. Knowing this, we can make changes to our lifestyle, the food we eat and how we manage stress to improve our skin health from within.

1. Nutrition is the first step in your skincare routine.

2. The food and drink we consume supply our skin with the nutrients it needs for health.

3. Our skin is intimately linked to our internal health; in fact, changes in the skin can be the only symptom of an underlying health condition.

4. Skin concerns, such as loss of radiance, acne and eczema arise as a combination of genetics (nature) and our lifestyle (nurture).

5. The 4-Step Skin Solution is designed to be easily adaptable and to deliver results, no matter what the skin concern might be.

STEP 1

Nutrition for Skin Health

2

Nutrients that Nourish, from A to Zinc

I have a confession to make: I used to take at least fifteen different vitamins a day in my twenties. I was convinced that the more I took, the healthier I would be. From multivitamins to selenium, every morning without fail I took a fistful of supplements. How did I end up with an expensive supplement habit? As I explained earlier, life as a junior doctor was tough, the days were long and busy; I survived on cafeteria food and snacked on chocolate bars, crisps and microwave ready meals. I thought that taking vitamins would be a shortcut to health and that in some way I was outsmarting my body. But it wasn't working. I was exhausted, struggling with energy slumps – and my uneven, washed-out skin paid the price.

Learning about nutrition transformed my approach to supplements. I've come to appreciate the variety, complexity and importance of vitamins contained in real food, and as a result I now take fewer supplements than ever. Although vitamin supplements can certainly be helpful in specific situations, my approach is firmly food first.

Supplements are so named for a reason. They shouldn't be seen as a shortcut to, or a substitute for, a healthy, balanced diet, but they can be used instead to replace or boost specific vitamins that may not be easily accessible through diet alone. Vitamin supplements contain individual nutrients, such as vitamins E and C, but real food is far more complex. Let's take the humble red pepper, for example: it contains over twenty different vitamins and minerals, in addition to fibre, carbohydrates and even a little protein. You'd struggle to achieve this complexity in a pill.

The effect of nutrition on our skin, hair and nails

Without a doubt, good nutrition is a requirement for skin health. When we lack certain nutrients, it's our skin, hair and nails that first show the signs of a deficiency. This principle is one of the topics that I teach to nutrition and dietetics students at King's College, London and it's an important aspect of understanding the complex relationship between food and skin health.

Occasionally in the clinic I see cases of nutrient deficiencies that are severe enough that they begin to affect the body, as we'll see with Priya's case below. But what we eat can have a huge impact on our overall appearance by helping to prevent and address deficiencies.

CASE STUDY: A LACK OF IRON

Priya was a mother of two, trying to juggle raising a family with a busy job in IT. She first noticed her hair loss while brushing her hair, but over a couple of months the rate of her hair shedding escalated and she began to notice clumps of hair falling out when she washed it. Priya's hair felt noticeably thinner, which led to a loss of confidence. Desperate to prevent further hair loss, she purchased a variety of hair tonics, shampoos and even hair supplements, but nothing seemed to work.

When Priya came to see me, she was despairing and tearful. When I examined Priya's hair it was dull and brittle with noticeable thinning. She had noticed that her hair loss seemed to slowly worsen after each of her pregnancies, but it had got to a point where it was very noticeable. I suspected her iron levels – one of the most important nutrients for hair health – had slowly dwindled over time, particularly as a result of her pregnancies. We performed simple blood tests to assess levels of iron and other nutrients in her blood, and the results were unsurprising: Priya's active iron levels (ferritin) were well below the healthy range, and she had developed mild anaemia. This explained both her tiredness and hair loss.

Together, we worked on how to improve her symptoms through a combination of diet and prescription supplements. Although I always recommend a food-first approach to meeting our nutritional requirements, in certain situations, particularly when there is a measurable deficiency causing symptoms, the fastest way to remedy the imbalance is through supplements. I advised Priya to include plant-based iron-rich foods (her preference), such as beans, lentils and green leafy vegetables, in her meals on a daily basis and to make sure that she included a good source of vitamin C (such as fresh lemon juice), which helps iron to be absorbed from the gut. When Priya returned to see me again three months later, she was relieved that her hair had stopped shedding and was starting to grow back, regaining a healthy sheen.

Nutrients for our skin

Priya's case demonstrates how deficiency in a single nutrient can have a profound impact on our skin and hair. For our overall health we need a combination of important nutrients in our diet. Before we can dive into what we need, let's take a step back and understand what makes up the food we eat. All food is made up of combinations of different nutrients, just like the red pepper I mentioned earlier.

We group nutrients into broad categories: macronutrients (protein, carbohydrates and fats) and micronutrients (vitamins and minerals).

Macronutrients

Protein, carbohydrates and fats are the building blocks that make up all the foods we eat.

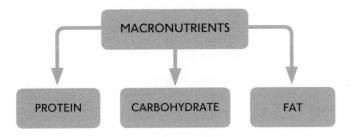

The macronutrients found in food.

An avocado, for example, contains mainly fats and carbohydrates, and a little protein. A piece of chicken breast is predominantly made up of protein with smaller amounts of carbohydrates and fats. Even though the ratios of each macronutrient vary between foods, the basic components remain the same.

All three macronutrients are required for our health, and we should aim to eat adequate amounts of each on a daily basis. In recent years, diets that exclude individual macronutrients have grown in popularity, including low-carbohydrate diets such as the keto diet, and very low-fat diets, but each macronutrient has its own unique benefits, and I believe that the combination of all three is critical for our health.

Diet trends – skin friend or foe?

Cutting carbs has been a huge dietary trend over the last decade, thanks to the Atkins diet and more recently the keto diet. In recent years, I've come across many patients who have tried the keto diet to improve their ▶

skin with mixed results. Such diets involve cutting out starches, including whole grains and even fruits and some vegetables, and often increasing the proportion of fats. The amount of carbs that you can eat on these diets is minimal and varies from about 15g to 40g net per day: the equivalent of one banana. The recommended fat intake is not restricted to what we consider to be good fats which I will describe later, but can include all fats, such as butter and cream. In fact, in the keto diet the majority of calories (70–80 per cent) are obtained from fat.

Cutting out carbohydrates means excluding most fruits, legumes (beans and pulses) and whole grains, such as brown rice and oats. It's easy to forget that these foods contain some of the highest levels of vitamins, minerals and fibre. Fibre is crucial, as it feeds our all-important gut bacteria, improving the absorption of nutrients, acts as an anti-inflammatory, and it can even reduce your chances of developing bowel cancer. Fibre in food also helps us to feel full and satiated.

Keto diets can also cause a very itchy rash to develop on the body, known simply as 'keto rash'. It is a direct result of skipping carbs, which causes the skin to become inflamed and triggers red bumps and blotches to appear. The treatment is simple: reintroduce carbohydrates into the diet, usually greater than 50g per day, and the rash disappears.

Most importantly, studies have shown that low-carbohydrate diets are no more effective than low-calorie diets when it comes to weight loss, so you're putting your body under unnecessary strain for minimal reward. Cutting out entire food groups is something that I never encourage, and that sits uneasy with me, as it can trigger restrictive eating habits and encourage feelings of guilt and shame around food.

The building blocks – as easy as 1, 2, 3

The proteins, carbohydrates and fats in the food we eat are broken down and digested in the gut. From here, they are absorbed into the bloodstream and distributed throughout the body where they are used for energy, repair and growth.

Proteins

Protein is essential for the repair and maintenance of all tissues and organs in the body, including the skin, so we need to ensure that we are consuming enough of it. Proteins present in the foods we eat are made up of individual amino acids that are strung together to form chains. Our digestive system breaks down these chains into individual amino acids that are then absorbed by the body. Amino acids are divided into those that are 'essential', which we can *only* obtain through foods, and those that are 'non-essential', which our body can make from other amino acids. After digestion, amino acids are absorbed and enter blood circulation, eventually making their way to the dermis (the deeper layer of the skin). Here they promote skin cell renewal and repair, and aid the production of fresh new skin cells. Amino acids are the raw materials needed to make structural proteins, such as collagen and elastin, which give our skin strength and elasticity. Protein is particularly important in recovery and for scar healing; for example, following surgery, cosmetic procedures or with acne scarring.

A lack of dietary protein can affect the skin, hair and nails, causing thinning and poor wound healing. It is important to remember that in order to meet our protein requirements we need to eat a variety of different protein sources, as each type contains a different combination of those all-important amino acids.

Meat, fish, quinoa and soya are rich sources of complete proteins, which means that they contain all the essential amino acids that are needed for health.

Complete Proteins	Incomplete Proteins
Fish	Nuts and seeds
Poultry and other meats	Lentils
Eggs	Whole grains
Dairy products	Legumes (lentils, peas and beans)
Quinoa	
Tofu and soya products	
Buckwheat	
Hempseed	

Vegetarians and vegans can more than meet their daily protein requirements by eating both plant-based complete proteins and combining incomplete proteins in their diet. Variety is the key here, as the different protein sources help us to reach our daily amino acid requirements. Aim to focus on nuts, seeds and legumes, such as black beans and chickpeas as well as soya products. On average, we require a minimum of 0.75g of protein per 1kg of body weight per day (this is the protein element of the food we eat, not the weight of protein food itself), although this varies considerably depending on our stage of life, level of activity and other factors.

We will find protein added to everything nowadays, including shakes, cereals and snack bars. We are bombarded with information telling us that we should be consuming more protein, but most of us should have no problem meeting our protein needs through food. Try experimenting with the types of protein-rich foods you eat. Increase the amount of peas, beans or lentils as an alternative to meat, for example; these foods have added health benefits as they contain phytonutrients and fibre. We will discuss easy ways to incorporate wholegrain fibre into your diet in Chapter 4.

Carbohydrates

Carbohydrates have gained a reputation for being inherently bad for you, and you'll often find advice suggesting that they should be cut out entirely, but that couldn't be further from the truth. Good carbs are an important part of a healthy diet, which is why they are a cornerstone of the SkinFood approach that I have devised.

Carbohydrates can be divided into two groups: simple and complex. Simple carbohydrates are made up of simple sugars such as glucose, fructose and galactose, also known as monosaccharides, whereas sugars such as sucrose, lactose and maltose are made up of pairs of simple sugars and are known as di-saccharides. Complex carbohydrates are chains of individual sugars and include starch and fibre. Our daily requirements for carbohydrates vary depending on our individual activity levels and body weight.

The reason why you've probably been told time and time again that sweets and candy are bad for you is because they contain primarily simple sugars and lack other nutrients. They also cause a rapid rise in blood sugar. On the other hand, sugars found in an apple, for example, are bound up with fibre and other nutrients. This means that they're released into the bloodstream at a slower rate and are much less likely to cause a blood sugar spike. The sugar in an apple is also eventually digested into simple sugars, but the rate at which this happens is much slower – plus you get all the benefits of added nutrients in the apple, such as fibre, vitamin C and antioxidants.

The glycaemic index

One way of categorising carbohydrates is the glycaemic index (GI). The index, which ranges from 0 to 100, represents the increase in blood sugar level that occurs when you eat a given food (for comparison, white table sugar scores 100 on the scale, whereas a pear has a score of 33).[1] Foods such as cakes, biscuits, sweets and refined carbohydrates such as white bread generally have a higher glycaemic index, whereas lower GI carbohydrates can be found in a variety of whole grains, vegetables and fruits.

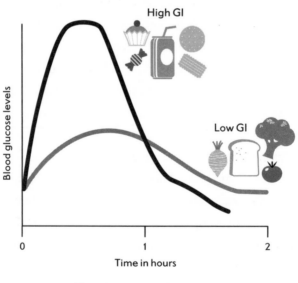

The glycaemic index graph.

There are many factors that affect how your blood sugar rises after you eat, including how ripe the fruit or vegetables are and how they have been prepared. In fact, fascinating research from my colleagues at King's College has demonstrated that there are unique factors that influence how each of us responds to the very same foods, including sugar. For example, my blood sugar response to a biscuit may vary markedly from a friend's and this will impact the types of food that are best for us. These important findings from the PREDICT 1 study underpin the importance of personalised nutrition and are likely to be integral to how we manage many conditions in the future.[1] It is also necessary to consider how you combine the foods as part of a meal or snack. Eating potatoes with a protein source, such as a bean chilli, results in a much lower rise in blood sugar than just eating the potato alone. The way you cook food also matters. A raw carrot has a GI of 16, but boiling it releases its natural sugars, causing the GI to increase to around 40. This phenomenon occurs because sugars are partially broken down by cooking. But I don't recommend getting too hung up on specific numbers – being mindful of refined and processed sugars and incorporating a variety of fruits, vegetables and whole grains should be the aim.

How does this all link back to our skin? Well, sugar can impact our skin health in many ways.

- Sugar triggers the formation of AGEs (advanced glycation end products) in the skin. AGEs bind to collagen and elastin in the deeper layers of the skin and cause it to stiffen, leading to the early signs of skin ageing.[3] A diet high in refined sugar will quite literally 'AGE' you!
- A high-GI diet may also cause acne flare-ups for some

people. We believe this is because high-GI foods can
cause surges in hormones, which worsen breakouts.

- Diets high in refined sugar can also negatively impact
gut health, which is linked to skin health.
- Excess refined sugars may also promote inflammation
in the body, and we know that inflammation is a
feature of many common skin concerns.

What then can we do? We all know that 4 o'clock feeling well:
you've hit a mid-afternoon standstill and you're desperate for a
few biscuits or some cake to perk you up. The quick sugar hit
will provide temporary relief, but the sugar slump that often
follows will leave you feeling lethargic and sluggish. In order
to combat this, we want to keep our blood sugar levels stable
throughout the day to feel our best so that we can say goodbye
to the afternoon blues. This is one of the primary aims of my
SkinFood approach. By combining proteins, carbohydrates and
healthy fats, your blood sugar stays nice and even. This is great
for skin health but, as an aside, having an even blood sugar helps
you to feel brighter and have more energy too.

Fats

Good fats are pivotal to skin and hair health, but many of us are
terrified by the idea of consuming fats, and we try to avoid them
at all cost. Although it's true that some types of fat aren't optimal
for health, we need to change gear and focus on including the
right types of fat in our diet. Healthy fats have an important role
in health. They can also help to protect us from heart disease,
depression and even certain cancers, so I'm sure the question on
your lips is: which fats are good fats?

Fats can broadly be divided up into two groups: saturated

and unsaturated. In general, it's the saturated fats that we need to moderate, as consuming these in excess has been linked to an increased risk of heart disease and stroke. You'll find this type of fat primarily in red meat, dairy products such as cheese and some plant-sourced oils such as palm oil and coconut oil. There is no need to demonise these foods, and it's fine to include them in sensible amounts in your diet, should you wish.

Healthy fats include monounsaturated fats found in avocados, nuts and olive oil, and polyunsaturated fats such as omega-3, which can be found in oily fish, walnuts and flaxseeds. Foods containing good fats should be eaten on a daily basis; we look at delicious ways to do this in the recipes in Chapter 10.

Omega-3 fatty acids, also known as essential fatty acids, are critical in maintaining healthy skin moisture levels, supporting the skin barrier function, reducing inflammation and promoting wound healing. In fact, omega-3 acids contribute to the natural oils produced in the skin, which offer smoothing and softening benefits by coating the outer layer of the skin and preventing moisture loss.[4] The body, however, is not capable of producing omega-3 on its own, so you need to ensure that your daily diet includes foods that are naturally rich in these fats; I like to refer to this as moisturising from within. In rare cases where you don't consume adequate essential fats, you can develop what's known as 'essential fatty acid deficiency', which causes severely dry, flaky skin and increased moisture loss. Although this is an extreme example, I cannot stress enough how optimising your intake of omega-3 is one of the most important nutritional changes you can make to support supple healthy skin.

The good news is that the benefits of omega-3 don't just stop at our skin. There has also been a great deal of research into its importance for our overall health, from our heart to our brain. Findings have shown that omega-3 may also have a positive effect on a number of conditions including depression, cancer, heart health and cholesterol.

Omega 3 is made up of three different types of fatty acids: EPA, DHA and ALA. EPA and DHA are found in food sources such as oily fish and other seafoods, while ALA is primarily found in plant-based foods such as nuts and seeds (for example walnuts and flaxseeds). ALA needs to be converted into EPA and DHA before it can be used in the body. As this process isn't completely efficient, it can be more challenging to obtain adequate omega-3 solely from a vegetarian or vegan diet.

How much omega-3 do we actually need? There aren't official intake guidelines in the UK, but studies show that we should be aiming for around 500µg of EPA and DHA daily, which approximately equates to one or two salmon fillets per week.[5] Where appropriate, I recommend omega-3 supplements to my patients, particularly those who don't eat oily fish or who follow a plant-based diet (omega-3 supplements derived from algae are now widely available). Like all supplements, you have to be careful how much you take, and if you're on medication, check with your doctor first, as they can interfere with drugs such as blood-thinners.

Omega-6 fatty acids, also known as linoleic acid, is another essential fatty acid found in plant oils and seeds such as sunflower oil and pumpkin seeds. As omega-6 is easily found in many foods, the vast majority of us should be able to meet our daily requirements through diet alone. Instead of considering supplementing, I would focus on improving the balance between omega-3 and omega-6 by increasing your intake of foods rich in omega-3.

Micronutrients

Micronutrients are vitamins and minerals that your skin (and the rest of your body) need to function well and stay in good health. We don't require huge quantities of each, but variety is important and – you've guessed it – the best way to ensure you're getting a nice mix of micronutrients is from a balanced diet.

Micronutrients from our diet are essential to the health of our skin, hair and nails, but did you know that nutrients are also some of the most widely used ingredients in skincare products too?

Here are just a few examples:

Vitamin C is a key antioxidant in our diet and a popular skincare ingredient known for its brightening and antioxidant functions. It helps to reduce pigment production and quench free radicals caused by ultraviolet light that can damage collagen.

Zinc is an important ingredient in anti-dandruff shampoos and is also used in acne treatments for its anti-bacterial and anti-inflammatory properties.

Vitamin B3 (also known as niacinamide) is one of the most commonly used skincare ingredients, helping to protect and support the skin barrier while reducing inflammation. It also reduces oil production and calms redness, so it's helpful in the treatment of breakouts.

Vitamin A, also known as retinol or retinoids, is one of the best-studied skincare ingredients. When used in the right percentage and formulation, it can help tackle many signs of ageing by boosting cell turnover and improving collagen production.

Dermatologists will prescribe retinoids for the targeted treatment of acne, where it helps to reduce oil production and unclogs pores.

Vitamin E, also known as tocopherol, has been used for over 50 years in dermatology and is an important skincare ingredient in numerous cosmetic products. Like vitamin C, vitamin E targets free radicals to soften the harmful effects of UV light and pollution on our skin. It is also commonly used as a preservative in oil-based skincare products.

Vitamin D, also known as the 'sunshine vitamin', is used in creams and ointments to treat psoriasis.

Polyphenols such as resveratrol are powerful antioxidants that have led to the formation of new beauty companies that are dedicated to exploring and promoting its benefits. Extracted from the skin of grapes, these compounds have been shown to have potent antioxidant effects, again reducing the impact of free radicals on the skin.

(Later in the book we will explore how well these skincare nutrients can be absorbed into the skin through specific creams or lotions. Not all creams are created equal in this respect.)

Now that you're armed with this knowledge, have a look on your bathroom shelf and see how many products contain hidden nutrients. It should come as no surprise that you'll also find a lot of these nutrients on your plate too!

Vitamins

The vitamins A, D, E and K are fat-soluble vitamins, which means that they are absorbed in the gut only when accompanied by fat or oil. This is why you often see vitamin E and D sold as oil-filled capsules rather than tablets. Fat-soluble vitamins are unique because they are stored by the body when an excess is taken. By contrast, water-soluble vitamins (such as vitamins B and vitamin C) cannot be stored by the body. When we have too much, our body tries to clear out the excess by passing it into urine. (You can learn more about vitamins and minerals on both the NHS and British Dietetic Association webpages, see Resources.)

Vitamin A (fat soluble) As mentioned earlier, vitamin A (retinoic acid) is one of the most researched ingredients used in skincare, as it fights wrinkles, reduces breakouts and neutralises pigmentation. It also plays an important role in maintaining the integrity of our skin barrier, as well as regulating the skin immune system. It really is pretty incredible. That said, I wouldn't recommend immediately rushing to your local pharmacy to stock up on vitamin A supplements, as you can also experience side effects from taking too much, such as skin peeling and hair loss, and extreme deficiencies are incredibly rare. Adults in the UK require only 600ug for women and 700ug for men – but please bear in mind that vitamin A is harmful to unborn babies, so avoid taking supplements if you are pregnant or planning to become pregnant.

Foods rich in vitamin A include liver, cod liver oil, mackerel and salmon. You can also find it in dairy products such as butter, Cheddar cheese and animal products such as eggs. Plant-based sources of vitamin A are easy to find, as they'll often have a vibrant red, orange or yellow hue, such as carrots, red peppers, sweet potatoes, mangoes, papayas and apricots.

I don't recommend supplementing your diet with additional vitamin A, as your daily requirements can easily be met through your food intake. If you want to harness the benefits of vitamin A to help clear acne, I would suggest incorporating a retinol-based skincare product into your routine instead of taking additional supplements.

Vitamin D (fat soluble) has a unique relationship with the skin. Not only is it essential for many skin functions, but it is also made within the skin itself. Exposing our skin to sunlight results in the production of activated vitamin D through UVB light. It is often associated with healthy bones, but over the years I have become more and more interested in the importance of vitamin D when it comes to our skin, hair and nails.

Vitamin D has been shown to perform numerous key functions in the skin such as helping cells to divide and renew, fighting infections and supporting the normal function of the immune system, as well as promoting wound healing and tissue repair after injury. It's also key to hair-follicle function and supports normal hair growth and development. Without moderate levels of this wonder vitamin, many common skin and hair conditions – such as eczema, psoriasis, vitiligo, acne and warts, hair loss and auto-immune dysfunction – can be potentially aggravated.[6]

Sunlight and vitamin D

'Am I getting enough vitamin D if I wear sunscreen?'

We all know that sunscreen is one of the most effective ways to fight signs of ageing, but by blocking UV rays, does it stop us from getting enough vitamin D? The simple answer is no. According to a study published in the *British*

Journal of Dermatology,[7] our skin can still make enough vitamin D even if we're wearing sunscreen.

'Can sunlight alone provide a sufficient source of vitamin D?'

If you live in the UK, you should be able to meet your daily vitamin D needs with just 15 minutes of sun exposure per day in the summer over the face, arms and legs; however, it is recommended that we take supplements during the winter. Although it's possible to obtain vitamin D through foods such as eggs (especially the yolks), oily fish, red meat and fortified breakfast cereals (that is, those that have vitamins and minerals added), it's hard work trying to get enough of it solely through what's on our plate. Another thing to bear in mind is that anyone with a deeper skin tone, or who prefers to keep their skin covered, should make sure to supplement their vitamin D intake all year round to avoid deficiency.

'How should I supplement?'

During the winter months (October to March) it is recommended that all adults supplement 10µg (400IU) in the UK. This can be in the form of capsules or sprays, but look at the label to make sure that you are buying vitamin D3, the active form, rather than vitamin D2.

Age	Vitamin D dose
Up to 1 year (and not receiving 500ml formula per day)	8.5–10µg (micrograms) per day

One to 4 years of age	10μg per day (400 IU)
Older children if they are not outdoors or mostly covered up, or they have darker skin tone	10μg per day (400 IU)
Adults during winter months as a minimum (October to March) or year-round if you aren't exposing your skin to the sun or have a darker skin tone	10μg per day (400–1,000 IU)

How you take your vitamin D also matters, as it requires fat to be present in order for it to be properly absorbed. Therefore, I'd recommend taking it with a meal that contains some healthy fat such as avocado or olive oil. A study in the *Journal of Bone and Mineral Research*[8] found that taking vitamin D with dinner, the heaviest meal of the day, can improve absorption by up to 50 per cent compared to taking it on an empty stomach or with a smaller meal. This is because the meal ensures the optimum release of enzymes such as bile that aid the absorption of fat-soluble vitamins.

NOTE Everyone forgets to take their vitamins! Because vitamin D is stored in the body, you can take it just once a week if that's easier. Taking 4,000 IU once per week would meet your requirements.

Vitamin E (fat soluble) A well-established antioxidant, vitamin E has been used as a skincare ingredient for over 50 years because of its ability to protect our skin cells from the damaging free radicals caused by UV light.[9] It is also a component of sebum, the oil that our skin naturally produces to keep it moist and supple.

In the skin, vitamin E is the main oil-soluble antioxidant and forms our first line of defence by reducing inflammation in the skin and supporting wound healing.

When it comes to incorporating vitamin E into our diets, look to foods such as olive oil, avocado, nuts, salmon, fortified bread and egg yolks, which are all rich sources of this vitamin. Although, like other antioxidants, vitamin E is an important part of a skin-friendly diet, we don't require huge amounts of it to meet our daily needs, so there's no need to spend money on supplements, even if it feels like a tempting shortcut to make the most of its powerful skin benefits. Instead, I would look for skincare products that contain vitamin E, because you'll see more of an effect by using it topically.

The water-soluble vitamins B and C are critical for the skin, as deficiencies can lead to striking changes in your skin and hair. Although they are readily absorbed in the gut, they are not stored in the body, which means that we need to ensure we are consuming enough foods rich in these vitamins to meet our daily nutritional needs; however, don't overdo it when it comes to increasing your consumption, as any excess vitamins will be simply flushed out through your urine. I mention this because you might have noticed a growing trend for IV (intravenous) vitamin drips in shopping centres and beauty spas, which promise glowing, radiant skin. Although they do offer temporary hydration, the cocktail of vitamins they contain are likely to be water-soluble so any excess will be removed by the body – essentially what you're paying for is very expensive wee!

The B vitamins comprise a family of eight vitamins that support the function of energy-releasing enzymes in the body. They are numbered as follows:

B1 thiamine
B2 riboflavin
B3 niacin
B5 pantothenic acid
B6 pyridoxine
B7 biotin
B9 folic acid
B12 cobalamin

If you're wondering where B4, B8, B10 and B11 have disappeared to, it's because the B vitamins were numbered in the order they were discovered and these omitted substances are no longer considered to be true vitamins, as they are not essential for healthy growth and well-being.

B vitamins regulate energy levels, brain function and cell metabolism and are involved in countless processes in the body, but what role do they play when it comes to skin?

Vitamin B2 (riboflavin) (water soluble) This is found in eggs, meat and milk. Deficiency is relatively rare but can develop in anyone following a plant-based diet, in older persons or pregnant/lactating women. Tongue swelling and soreness can occur, and there is an increased frequency of seborrheic dermatitis: a scaly and greasy red rash found in the scalp and creases of the nose and brows.

Vitamin B3 (niacin) (water soluble) This vitamin is used to release energy within the cells through a series of reactions. Although a vitamin B3 deficiency is generally uncommon, I did come across it during my years working at the hospital. I once met a young girl who had severe inflammatory bowel disease, who had lost so much weight that she was practically bedbound. I had been called to see her because of a rash she had developed over her feet and around her mouth. I noticed a thick red scaly rash on her feet as well as cracks at the corners of her mouth – classic signs of severe vitamin B3 deficiency and also known as pellagra. Thankfully, supplementing her diet with vitamin B3 resulted in the rash disappearing within a week of treatment.

Studies have shown that we might be able to use a derivative of vitamin B3, known as nicotinamide, to prevent skin cancer. A leading medical journal, the *New England Journal of Medicine*,[10] explained how researchers had examined the efficacy of nicotinamide in preventing types of skin cancer known as non-melanoma skin cancer by carrying out a study on a group of participants who were at high risk of developing new skin cancers. The participants were given either a twice-daily dose of 500µg of nicotinamide or a placebo (or dummy drug). The results showed that those who had taken the supplements had reduced their risk of developing new skin cancers by 23 per cent compared to those who received the placebo.

How does a vitamin prevent skin cancer? Well, it is really quite remarkable. As you may already know, skin cancer can develop from exposure to sunlight, as the sun's UV rays trigger DNA damage that accrues over time and can ultimately lead to cancer. Nicotinamide, however, appears to boost cellular energy and promote DNA repair to combat damage caused by exposure to the sun. This doesn't mean that we can rely on nicotinamide and ditch the sunscreen. I cannot stress enough that protecting our skin from UV rays using SPF (sun-protection factor), seeking shade and covering up are the best forms of prevention, but nicotinamide could be an added benefit for anyone at higher risk of developing skin cancer.

You'll find B3 in many commonly consumed foods, including nuts, seeds, legumes, brown rice, bananas, fish, poultry and red meat.

Vitamin B5 (pantothenic acid) (water soluble) Vitamin B5 is required to maintain the protective skin barrier. It is converted into co-enzyme A, which helps to build the skin barrier and promote skin renewal (the continual process by which older skin cells are replaced by younger ones). You may be familiar with what's known as panthenol or pro-vitamin B5, as it's used in a variety of hair-care products to help soften and smooth your hair. There isn't much evidence at all to support taking B5 supplements, so my advice is to focus on obtaining it through dietary sources such as mushrooms, fish, avocadoes, eggs and lean chicken.

Vitamin B7 (biotin) (water soluble) is marketed, often in very high doses, as a costly hair loss supplement. Although a biotin deficiency can cause hair loss, weak nails and dry skin, it's a vitamin so commonly found in foods that developing a deficiency is actually incredibly rare. At present, there isn't enough evidence to justify the high doses of biotin (sometimes over ten times the recommended daily amount) that's sold in hair supplements.

Taking high doses of biotin can have other unwanted side effects, such as acne and breakouts, and it can also interfere with hormonal blood test results. Instead focus on including biotin-rich foods in your diet, such as egg yolks, legumes, sweet potatoes, nuts and seeds.

Vitamin B9 (folic acid) (water soluble) Folate deficiency most commonly affects pregnant and breastfeeding women, although it can also occur in people with bowel inflammation or in the elderly. Symptoms include fatigue, weakness and nausea or diarrhoea. It can be linked to a sore red tongue, mouth ulcers and sores at the corners of the mouth – and in rare cases it can cause red peeling skin. Although I do check folate levels in my patients, I rarely find deficiencies that require treatment. This is because folate is found in a wide variety of foods, and many prepared foods such as cereal and bread are already fortified with folate.

Vitamin B12 (cobalamin) (water soluble) plays a role in metabolism and DNA quality, as well as red blood-cell formation. It's important to know that it's the only vitamin exclusively found in animal products (meat, fish and dairy), so if you follow a vegan or vegetarian diet, I would recommend regularly taking a B12 supplement. I have seen plant-based patients who have developed a B12 deficiency that's led to symptoms such as a sore tongue, mouth ulcers and areas of darker skin pigmentation. Some people with gut issues may not absorb vitamin B12 well, so they can also become deficient. Low levels of B12 can also contribute to hair shedding. If you're experiencing any symptoms, do go to see your doctor, as it's easy to check your vitamin B12 levels with a simple blood test, so there's no need to worry.

Vitamin C (water soluble) Known as the gold-standard antioxidant, vitamin C is one of the most readily available vitamins, both in our skincare and in supplements. For many years, high-strength vitamin C has been recommended for all manner of concerns from fighting coughs and colds to reducing cancer risk, but many of these claims cannot be backed up with science. With regard to the skin, however, vitamin C really is the queen of antioxidants. It rapidly quenches free radicals to prevent the

UV- and pollution-induced damage that leads to premature ageing and hyperpigmentation. It also helps wounds to heal, supports our immune system and helps to make hormones, including those that regulate stress, in the brain and nerves. It's pretty miraculous.

As well as being a powerhouse antioxidant, vitamin C promotes collagen production and is critical in the protein's formation, as it helps to stabilise its coil-shaped structure so that it retains its shape, which is key for maintaining plump skin. In a study in children who had experienced burns, the participants who were given vitamin C and E showed improved healing compared to those who hadn't taken supplements.[11] The reason why vitamin C plays such a profound role in wound healing is because fibroblast cells, which are responsible for the production of collagen in the dermis, are highly dependent on vitamin C. If you suffer from acne scarring, or you're thinking about having a cosmetic procedure such as laser or a chemical peel, try to incorporate more vitamin C-rich foods into your diet or consider taking supplements to support skin recovery.

It's worth bearing in mind that, as with almost all vitamins, our body can't make vitamin C, so ensuring that you get your daily intake through your diet and supplementation is vital. The richest sources of vitamin C come from fresh fruits – especially citrus fruits – and vegetables such as red peppers. Vitamin C deficiency is rare, but it has noticeable effects on the skin. It can cause roughened hair follicles, bleeding and bruising (think sailors in the past and scurvy). Unsurprisingly, a lack of vitamin C also slows down the wound-healing process due to diminished collagen production. That being said, vitamin C deficiency, or scurvy, has become almost obsolete, but it emphasises how critical vitamin C is for skin health.

'How should I supplement?'

The question really comes down to this: is more necessarily better? There is a trend known as mega-dosing that encourages taking several thousand milligrams of vitamin C per day. Although this might sound like a good idea, our gut lining has a limited ability to absorb vitamin C and this drops with dosages greater than 1,000µg. Research has also shown that in very high doses, vitamin C can switch from *anti*oxidant to *pro*oxidant and actually accelerate tissue damage rather than protecting against it.

The different forms of vitamin C

When it comes to vitamin C supplementation, things can get confusing. There are numerous types of vitamin C available, including ascorbic acid, mineral ascorbates, time-release vitamin C, esterified vitamin C and liposomal vitamin C. Man-made ascorbic acid appears to be equivalent to the naturally occurring form found in foods such as orange juice and broccoli, with studies so far not demonstrating superiority of one particular type over another. From my study of the literature, the liposomal form of vitamin C shows some strengths over standard vitamin C. By encapsulating vitamin C – essentially surrounding it in a bubble of lipids (fats) – the gut can more readily absorb the vitamin. We are lacking independent studies that show clear skin benefits of liposomal vitamin C, but the limited evidence available is positive so far. It is certainly something worth trying if you are looking to improve collagen, elasticity and protect against environmental stressors, but stick to a dose of 1,000µg or less per day.

Minerals for skin health

Zinc is a mineral required for many processes in the body. Low zinc levels can cause dry, cracked skin, affect hair growth and lead to nail abnormalities. How then can we make sure that we're getting enough zinc in our diet? Foods rich in this mineral include red meat, poultry and shellfish, as well as fortified foods (such as breakfast cereals) and pulses. If your diet is totally plant-based, you're at a higher risk of developing a zinc deficiency. A component called phytic acid, found in whole wheat, legumes and whole grains can interfere with the absorption of zinc from the gut so be mindful of this. If your diet is lacking in zinc-rich foods and you are struggling to incorporate them into your meals, you can consider taking a low supplement dose of 15µg per day. It's worth bearing in mind that more is not always better; in fact, excessive zinc supplementation can lead to unwanted side effects such as nausea and occasionally stomach cramps.

Selenium You'll very often find selenium in hair, skin and nail supplements, but you actually need only a very small amount of selenium in your diet to meet your requirements. In the skin, selenium functions as an antioxidant to prevent free-radical damage and premature skin ageing. In addition, it is required for thyroid function, heart health and immune responses as well as brain health. Both high and low levels of selenium can prove problematic. In excess it can actually contribute to hair loss, so check your supplement and make sure you aren't taking more than the recommended daily amount.

Brazil and cashew nuts are rich in selenium, as are fortified cereals, chicken and shellfish; however, this isn't your signal to go off and enjoy a large bag of Brazil nuts, as eating several a day can actually result in excess selenium intake. A single large Brazil nut contains 90mcg, easily exceeding your daily requirement of 25–50mcg per day.

Overall, unless you have been diagnosed with a selenium deficiency, this is a supplement you can skip. It's relatively easy to meet your selenium requirements through diet, so there's no need to splash out on additional supplementation.

Iron As we saw from Priya's story in the case study on page 53, iron is vital for hair health. I am almost obsessive about checking iron levels in my clinic, because many women aren't aware that they're suffering from low iron levels and experience dry, itchy skin and hair loss. The symptoms can be subtle and progress slowly over many months or even years. Iron is a vital nutrient, incorporated into red blood cells, and it is this that allows them to transport oxygen around the body. When iron levels fall, our bodies cannot make enough red blood cells, and this can lead to anaemia as well as symptoms such as fatigue and breathlessness.

Causes, symptoms and signs of low iron

Iron deficiency is incredibly common – in fact it is one of the most common nutritional deficiencies in the world, so it's important to be aware of some of the causes and symptoms.

The causes of low iron

- Inadequate iron in the diet
- Pregnancy and breastfeeding
- Heavy periods
- Blood loss from other causes
- Inflammation in the bowel
- Chronic illnesses

The symptoms of low iron levels

- Fatigue
- Shortness of breath
- Palpitations
- Cold hands and feet

The signs of low iron in your skin and nails

- Brittle nails, spoon-shaped nails (also known as koilonychia)
- Premature grey hairs
- Pale skin
- Dry, brittle hair
- Hair loss
- Dry itchy skin
- Sores and cracks on either side of the mouth

Many women of childbearing age can suffer from low iron and anaemia caused by their periods and pregnancy. In a study of premenopausal women, the single most common cause of hair loss was anaemia resulting from low iron levels.[12] If you have symptoms of an iron deficiency or persistent hair loss, I would advise seeing your doctor or dermatologist to check your levels of iron, and the active protein which stores it, ferritin (among other tests) to see if insufficient iron might be the root cause.

How to boost iron Iron in food can be divided into two groups: haem iron and non-haem iron. Haem iron is derived from haemoglobin and is found in animal proteins such as red meat, poultry and seafood. It is the most easily absorbed type of iron, but in general, we need to be cautious with the amount of red meat we eat as excess is linked to long-term health conditions.[13] Non-haem iron is found in plant sources such as leafy green vegetables, and is more difficult for the body to absorb. It is certainly possible to meet your daily iron needs on a vegetarian or vegan diet, but it takes a little bit more planning. I would recommend focusing on beans, dark-green leafy vegetables (such as kale), iron-fortified cereals and breads, and dried fruits such as raisins and apricots.

Iron is fickle, as it isn't easily absorbed in the gut, particularly when combined with certain foods; for example, compounds in tea and coffee, and the calcium found in dairy products, can interfere with adequate iron absorption. My advice is to pair iron-rich foods with vitamin C to maximise how much you absorb, with some studies showing that doing this can allow you to absorb up to four times more iron.

> ## Tips to improve your iron intake
>
> - Combine kale or spinach (cooked or raw) with lemon juice rather than creamy sauces to avoid dairy.
> - Enjoy iron-fortified cereals with non-dairy milk, some dried fruit combined with strawberries.
> - Eat oranges or satsumas paired with a handful of nuts.

Iron supplements There are a multitude of iron supplements available, from tablets to liquids and sprays. You might be overwhelmed by the volume of choice and unsure where to start, but it all depends on how low your iron levels are. For iron-deficiency anaemia confirmed on blood tests, I usually recommend prescription-strength supplements; however, if you are just looking to top up your iron levels because you think you might not be getting enough in your diet, over-the-counter supplements should be enough. Be aware, however, that iron supplements can cause constipation. The recommended daily allowance in the UK is 15μg per day, which can be in tablet, liquid or spray form depending on your preference.

Specific considerations for vegetarian and vegan diets

Vegetarian and vegan diets offer a number of benefits and we should all aim to eat a greater variety of fruits and vegetables; however, certain nutrients are a little trickier to obtain from plants alone. As we have seen, hair health can be affected by nutrient deficiencies, and more recent studies have also indicated that following a predominantly plant-based diet may result in slower wound healing after cosmetic procedures.[14]

If you are vegan or vegetarian, it's important to ensure that you're getting enough of certain vitamins that are mainly found in animal products, in your diet. But don't worry, there are several ways you can do this:

Vitamin B12 Check the labels of fortified cereals and some non-dairy milks, as many of these will contain added B12.

- I am a big fan of nutritional yeast, which has a cheesy, nutty flavour while being completely vegan and frequently fortified in B12 (be sure to check the package before buying). Two teaspoons per day is often adequate to meet your daily requirement for B12, but brands vary, so be sure to check the label.
- If you would prefer to go for supplementation instead, that's fine too. Look for cyanocobalamin, the most stable form of B12, and the Vegan Society in the UK recommends a daily dose of 10mcg.

Omega-3 As mentioned earlier, it is harder to achieve your daily requirements of omega-3 fats through a vegan or vegetarian diet alone. Although flaxseeds, walnuts and hemp seed oil all contain omega-3, I would also recommend supplementation with vegan omega-3 at a dose of 500µg EPA/DHA per day.

Iron As we have seen, non-haem iron is found in plant-based foods and is less easily absorbed than haem iron from meat and fish. Therefore, if you are vegan or vegetarian, you will need to consume higher amounts of dietary iron to meet requirements.

You'll find iron in foods such as spinach, kale, lentils, tofu and even nuts. Pair with vitamin C-rich foods to promote absorption. If you have any signs of low iron (see page 80), experience heavier periods, or are pregnant or breastfeeding, you might benefit from taking a daily iron supplement as well. I would, however, suggest checking with your doctor first.

Protein Plant-based proteins can be found in a huge variety of different foods, including soya, quinoa, beans, pulses and even brown rice. It requires thought and planning, but you can easily meet your daily requirements through diet alone. If you are aiming to build muscle and undertake weight-training, plant-based protein supplements (such as pea- or brown rice-based) may be worth considering.

The SkinFood guide to supplements

Hopefully the information that I've shared so far will have helped you to make a decision on whether you might need to incorporate supplements into your diet. If you're still undecided or need a refresher, the table below is designed as a quick reference guide on when to go ahead and supplement, and the dosage you'll need to take.

Vitamin/ nutrient	When do you need to take it?	Dose range
Omega-3	If you don't eat oily fish at least twice per week or are vegan/vegetarian	500µg EPA/DHA fish or algae-derived omega-3

Iron	If you have symptoms of low iron, have your levels checked with your doctor. If you are vegan or vegetarian and have difficulty meeting your needs through diet alone	15µg daily is the recommended amount for women between 19 and 50 years but this could be higher if your levels are low. Take alongside vitamin C (either a small glass of orange juice or a supplement) to maximise absorption
Vitamin D	We should all take vitamin D during the winter months (October to March) and also in the summer if you have darker skin or don't get much sun	400–1,000 IU daily
B12	If you are vegan or vegetarian, it is recommended to take vitamin B12, as this is primarily found in animal products	10 mcg daily
Vitamin C	Not everyone needs a vitamin C supplement, but it can help to support wound healing (such as acne scars or following cosmetic procedures). It may also help with wrinkle prevention and it supports collagen formation	500–1,000µg per day, ideally liposomal vitamin C. This can be taken for a one-month trial to see if you notice an improvement

Key skin-friendly takeaways

1. Our skin requires a balance of nutrients for health.

2. In most cases, we can achieve this through a balanced diet, which includes protein, carbohydrates and healthy fats.

3. Supplementing specific vitamins and minerals can be helpful in certain situations.

4. Low iron is a common cause of hair loss and dry itchy skin.

5. Low vitamin D levels can play a role in many different skin conditions.

6. Good fats such as omega-3 are key for skin health.

3

The Gut–Skin Connection

Now that we have an understanding of the vitamins and minerals that contribute to healthy skin, it's time to delve deeper into the unique relationship between nutrition and skin health. To do this we need to turn our attention to our gut – and the fascinating world of the gut microbiome, which is now widely considered the epicentre of human health; but first things first: what exactly is the gut microbiome?

The gut is home to trillions of microorganisms (bacteria, fungi and viruses) that are collectively known as the gut microbiome (GM). In fact, there are over ten times the number of microbe cells in our gut than human cells in our entire body, and the gut microbiome itself weighs about 2kg.

Over the last decade, an explosion of ground-breaking research in the field of gut health has allowed us to discover more and more about how these bugs shape who we are.[1] Over 1,000 species of bacteria have been identified in the gut, and they have been linked to every aspect of our health, from depression to weight issues and, of course, our skin health. The exciting news is that we have the power to influence our gut microbes directly through the foods we eat. There are two key characteristics that make for a healthy gut microbiome:

1　Balance: having plenty of 'good' gut bacteria, as opposed to the less beneficial 'bad' bacteria.
2　Diversity: having a variety of different species of good bacteria in the gut.

'How do I know if I have a "good" gut microbiome?'

You might be thinking that we can't see our gut microbiome, so how do we know if we have enough 'good' gut microbes? Well, there are lots of indicators that will show whether your gut is working properly:

- A smooth, sausage-shaped bowel movement that sinks to the bottom of the toilet.
- Bowel movements should be painless and strainless.
- You don't have excessive wind or bloating.
- Food you've eaten passes through the gut in about a day.
- Although there aren't firm rules here, bowel movements should be somewhere between three times per day and three times per week.

Finding balance

The balance between good and bad bacteria in the gut is essential to our overall well-being. Good bacteria (such as *Lactobacillus acidophilus* and *Bifidobacterium bifidum*) perform many roles:

- Help to digest food and absorb nutrients.
- Help to make vitamins such as folic acid, vitamins B6 and B12.
- Keep the levels of bad bacteria low.
- Help to protect the lining of the intestinal wall barrier.
- Help to regulate the immune system to reduce unwanted inflammation.

An excess of bad bacteria (such as *Escherichia coli* and *Bacteroides fragilis*), on the other hand, can have adverse effects on your health and contribute to inflammation. We call this imbalance dysbiosis, and it has been linked to several common skin conditions such as acne, rosacea, eczema and psoriasis. Genetics, certain health conditions and lifestyle factors can influence the composition of our gut microbiome, but the most powerful thing we can do to improve our GM is to make conscious tweaks to our diet: good bacteria need food to survive, and what they love best is fibre, which we know is found mainly in whole grains, fruits and vegetables. We will look at further ways to support gut health through our diet shortly.

Although we are still discovering how imbalances in the GM contribute to skin inflammation, there are several theories. For example, good bacteria make beneficial anti-inflammatory compounds called short-chain fatty acids (SCFAs). These clever substances have a huge range of effects on the human body, such as reducing inflammation, controlling appetite and fighting certain cancers – and they contribute to skin health too.[1] In addition, the gut microbiome is partly responsible for training our immune system to work at its best, and this is important as, when out of balance, the immune system can cause unwanted inflammation that can take the form of skin conditions like eczema and psoriasis.

The leaky gut

Just as the skin has a barrier, the gut does too. Some suggest that when the gut barrier, a protective shield lining the gut from top to bottom, becomes inflamed, it becomes too permeable or 'leaky'. One theory is that this allows particles that should usually remain within the gut to escape into the bloodstream, triggering inflammation and exacerbating a broad range of skin conditions. The often-proposed solution to this problem is to cut out gluten and dairy. But is there evidence to support this idea?

Looking at the research, the leaky gut theory appears somewhat exaggerated and oversimplified. It turns out that leakiness of the gut is a normal phenomenon, and it happens after we eat to allow nutrients from digested food to enter our bloodstream. In some gut conditions, such as coeliac disease and Crohn's disease, the gut barrier may not be working as effectively as it should do, however, due to inflammation and it then becomes too permeable as a result. Bad bacteria can also contribute to intestinal inflammation and increased permeability or leakiness.

Advocates of the leaky-gut theory will also often promise cures through special diets, such as drinking huge amounts of bone broth and taking supplements such as collagen to repair the gut lining. I've spoken to patients who have painstakingly boiled vats of bones for hours in an attempt to improve their skin health, but I personally haven't seen the benefits of this approach. Having scoured the scientific literature, I am afraid to say that I can't find evidence to back up this claim. If bone broth makes you feel good, by all means go ahead, but please don't assume that it will heal your gut or skin – spend your time (and money) elsewhere. Instead, try some of the science-backed ways of supporting your microbiome and protecting the gut lining that I share with you later in this chapter.

Probiotic supplements

The World Health Organization (WHO) defines probiotics as 'living microorganisms that confer a health benefit when administered in adequate amounts' – and this is a topic that frequently comes up in the clinic. Is it worth taking a probiotic and, if so, which one? Should you take a multi-strain probiotic or a single strain? Is more always better? I should start by saying that the best way to improve your gut microbiome is through the dietary advice described in Chapter 4. You could certainly consider adding a probiotic in addition to these measures, however.

Probiotics cover a huge range of different species of bacteria in different quantities. The reality is that we still don't yet have evidence to recommend specific probiotics reliably for most skin conditions. If you're looking for a comprehensive resource to understand probiotics, try the Clinical Guide to Probiotics Available in the US (usprobioticguide.com), which has collated research for many different health conditions. It discusses the different types of bacteria to look for, the dosage and how long to take something for; however, at the time of writing, skin conditions are not included in this guide, and this is largely because there aren't enough quality studies to confirm whether probiotics are helpful in treating skin complaints. That doesn't mean that they aren't worth trying, and I do recommend them in certain situations (which we'll come to very soon), so here are some tips to keep in mind when thinking about probiotics:

- How many bacteria? Look for five to ten billion colony-forming units (CFU).
- How many strains of bacteria does it contain? Again, more doesn't always mean better. The thing to look out for is whether the probiotic contains the right type of bacteria for the condition you are looking to treat.
- Has the probiotic been studied to ensure the bacteria reach the gut alive?
- Has the product been used in any clinical trials for the condition you are wanting to treat?
- If you have a weakened immune system, consult your doctor or dietitian before taking a probiotic.

If you want to try a probiotic, I would recommend taking them regularly for at least 3 months in order to see if there is any benefit. Below, we take a look at specific gut health advice for individual skin concerns.

The GM and acne

The driving force behind acne is increased sebum, blocked pores and inflammation, as we saw on page 29. Interestingly, research suggests that over half of all people with acne also experience imbalances in their gut microbiome. It's believed that the inflammation caused by the GM imbalance may contribute to acne, and there is some early research that suggests probiotics might have a positive effect on the skin. In one study, participants who took a specific probiotic alone for 12 weeks for their skin saw a 30 per cent reduction in acne lesions, inflammation and reduced sebum levels too.[3] As part of acne treatment, we might use antibiotics for several months at a time. In such cases I often recommend also taking a probiotic alongside in order to reduce the knock-on impact on the gut microbiome. Studies suggest that this can help to reduce side effects from medication and could also improve acne further.

The GM and ageing well

Our gut microbes are part of us and, as such, they age with us too, changing and maturing over the course of our lives. In fact, there are differing communities of bacteria present in our GM during childhood, adulthood and into our elderly years. The reality is that we all want to feel as good as we can for as long as possible, so in order to find out the secrets to healthy ageing, researchers have looked to those who do it better than anyone: centenarians. People who live to the age of 100 and above are remarkable, and how and why they outlive others has been a source of fascination for decades.

One theory is that the secret to their longevity is the gut microbiome. A higher abundance of microbes associated with good health, such as *Akkermansia*, *Bifidobacterium* and *Lactobacillus*, have been found in the GM of centenarians. Good bacteria have been shown to reduce inflammation and maintain the integrity of the intestines, suggesting a central role in both the immune system and ageing. Studies of people who live to an advanced age also show that they have greater microbe diversity.[4] Although we don't quite know yet whether a good gut microbiome helps us to stay looking young, it could certainly help us to feel our best for as long as possible.

The GM and rosacea

Rosacea was one of the first skin conditions linked to gut health. Research has shown that patients who suffer from rosacea have an increased chance of developing an overgrowth of *Helicobacter pylori*, a spiral-shaped bug found in the stomach. This can lead to a range of uncomfortable symptoms such as indigestion, heartburn, nausea and bloating. It is understood that *H. pylori* releases compounds that cause inflammation in the gut, which in turn trigger skin flushing.

More recently, rosacea has been potentially linked with another gut imbalance known as small intestinal bacterial overgrowth (SIBO). Although the majority of our gut bacteria should live in our large bowel (the thicker part of the intestine that leads to the anus), SIBO occurs when bugs travel up to the small bowel and cause symptoms such as bloating and feelings of fullness. Some studies have shown that SIBO is thirteen times more likely to occur in people with rosacea than those in the general population, and it's believed that gut inflammation may also contribute to skin redness and flushing.

Treating SIBO may help rosacea management. In one small study, 46 per cent of people with rosacea were also found to have SIBO. Treating SIBO with a 1-week course of antibiotics resulted in substantial improvements to patients' skin and rosacea symptoms;[5] when these patients were reviewed 3 years later, many of them remained with clear skin despite no additional treatment.[6]

In addition to SIBO and *H. pylori*, there are other digestive conditions that have also been linked to rosacea, including irritable bowel syndrome (IBS), inflammatory bowel disease (IBD) and coeliac disease (gluten allergy). As a result, if you have rosacea, it's important to check for gut symptoms. This is the personal checklist that I use:

- Ache or burning pain in tummy
- Nausea
- Loss of appetite
- Excessive burping
- Significant bloating and feelings of fullness
- Reflux or heartburn
- Diarrhoea or constipation

I am often asked about whether gluten should be avoided if you have rosacea. Current research has not identified gluten as being a trigger for rosacea, but some people find that their symptoms improve when they avoid gluten-containing foods, such as bread and pasta. This could point to another underlying gut condition such as those mentioned above, as some of these will benefit from a gluten-free diet.

Aim to support the balance of gut microbes through your diet if you have rosacea by consuming a wide variety of fruit and probiotic foods such as sauerkraut and kefir. If the histamine in these foods triggers a flare of rosacea, it is worth considering taking a probiotic for at least 3 months to support the GM. Be mindful when choosing a probiotic, as both *Lactobacillus casei* (excluding *Lactobacillus paracasei* 431) and *Lactobacillus bulgaricus* are high in histamines and could worsen symptoms. I would suggest trying a probiotic that includes *Lactobacillus rhamnosus GG* instead.

The GM and psoriasis

Research suggests that people with psoriasis may have less diverse gut bacteria and less good bacteria compared with those who don't. In a study to investigate the role of the GM in patients with psoriasis, scientists looked at the GM of 52 patients and made comparisons with healthy people. They observed differences, but one thing that stood out was that numbers of the friendly bacteria, *Akkermansia muciniphila*, were lower in those with psoriasis.[7] Other studies have also shown that patients with psoriasis have less diverse microbiomes in general, which, as we know, is another key marker of gut health. This makes sense, as we know that imbalances in our gut bacteria contribute to inflammation.

Research in this area is still in its early days, and we haven't quite figured out yet which bacteria are consistently altered in people with psoriasis; however, three separate small trials have shown that adding a probiotic supplement could significantly improve psoriasis and lower levels of inflammation in the skin.[8] In addition to boosting the gut microbiome through diet, you could try a good general probiotic for 3 months if you want to see whether it helps.

The GM and eczema

Studies in babies have shown that a reduced GM diversity at six months old is linked to a greater chance of developing eczema by the age of two. This finding has led to several clinical trials that have tested whether giving probiotics to babies might be helpful in preventing eczema.

Most of the studies conducted have explored the use of *Lactobacillus* and *Bifidobacterium* probiotics in children and adults, including during pregnancy, and the evidence is generally positive with results showing somewhat lowered rates of eczema in participants who took the probiotics. As a result, the World Allergy Organization recommends that pregnant women whose babies are at high risk of developing eczema (for example those who have close family members with eczema, asthma or food allergies) take a probiotic during pregnancy and while breast-feeding and that their baby should be given a probiotic until 6 months old.[9]

These experts argue that although the evidence supporting the use of probiotics is yet to be clinically proven, there is very little harm in taking them. In the clinic I recommend looking for the species *Lactobacillus rhamnosus GG*, for which there is some supportive evidence in eczema prevention in children. There are specific probiotics for pregnancy and for babies too, so do look out for these, and if this is a relevant concern, I would suggest also speaking with your doctor. However, studies are yet to demonstrate that probiotics help to improve established eczema in adults. If you're still curious about their effect, then you can consider trialling a probiotic containing *Lactobacillus rhamnosus GG* for three months, in addition to supporting your gut health through diet, to see if you notice any improvement.

The gut–brain–skin axis

Not only do the brain and gut communicate with the skin individually, but in fact all three organs are connected to one another. In the last few years, a new and exciting concept has emerged: the gut–brain–skin axis. Essentially, this describes how these three separate and distant organs influence one another. The illustration allows us to visualise how this relationship works.

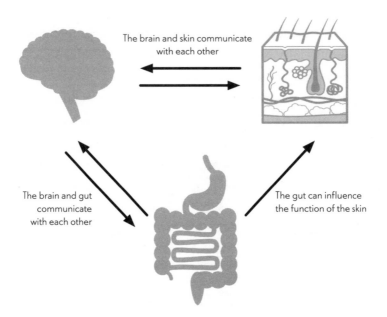

The gut, brain and skin are all interlinked and
constantly in communication with one another.

We now understand that our gut microbes can play a profound role in our mood – with the term 'gut feeling' taking on a whole new meaning. This is because the gut is responsible for producing hormones that affect our mood, most notably serotonin, the happy hormone. It's even thought that certain probiotics can act as mood enhancers by helping the gut to produce more serotonin.

As we will come to learn in Step 2, our mind and our mood can powerfully affect our skin. Stress is a major trigger for many skin conditions, so by supporting our gut microbiome, not only are we helping our skin health but our brain health too, which may in turn help to reduce the effect of stress on the skin. In essence we want everything to be working in harmony!

Your gut microbiome masterplan

In the same way that we can help our gut microbiome, we can also harm it. A diet high in processed foods, refined sugars and salt is notoriously problematic for gut microbiomes, as it reduces diversity and changes the balance in favour of bad bacteria. Other aspects of our lifestyle, such as smoking, excess alcohol, poor sleep and stress, can also have a negative impact on our gut health. But by making deliberate diet and lifestyle choices we are able to alter our gut microbes and improve diversity as well as the overall levels of good bacteria within weeks. My recommendation is that you start by taking the following simple steps to improve your gut health:

Eat a variety of plants (try to aim for thirty per week)

Eating a diverse and varied plant-rich diet is one of the first steps in supporting gut health. The different nutrients in each unique fruit and vegetable offers sustenance for the multiple types of good gut bacteria. The American Gut Project looked at the gut microbiome in a number of healthy adults and found that people who ate more than thirty different plant foods each week had a more diverse gut microbiome compared with those who ate ten or fewer.[10] Those who reached thirty or more also had more good bacteria that produce the anti-inflammatory short-chain fatty acids, which is one of the reasons why a plant-predominant diet is an anti-inflammatory one.

Although thirty plants may seem like a lot, it's easier than you think. This number isn't only restricted to fruit and vegetables, but it includes whole grains, oils, nuts, seeds and spices as well as coffee, tea, herbs and plain chocolate. If you want to get started straight away, you can turn to Chapter 10 for easy and delicious recipes to boost your gut microbiome.

Include **pro**biotic- and **pre**biotic-rich foods in your diet

As we know, good gut bacteria reduce inflammation and reinforce the gut barrier, but in order to carry out these important functions they need food to survive – and what they love to feast on the most is fibre. Probiotic foods are those that *contain* good bacteria, whereas prebiotics are a specific type of indigestible fibre that acts as fertiliser for the good gut bacteria. These fibres include inulin, fructooligosaccharides (FOS) and galactooligosaccharides (GOS).

Here are some examples of prebiotic-rich foods:

Apples
Asparagus
Bananas
Barley
Dried figs and mangoes
Fennel
Flaxseeds
Garlic
Jerusalem artichoke
Leeks
Nuts (hazelnuts, pistachio nuts, cashew nuts
and almonds)
Oats
Onions
Rye

As we have seen, prebiotics feed the good bacteria in our gut. Probiotic foods, such as live yoghurt or kefir, introduce additional good bacteria in the form of living bacteria or yeasts. Eating these on a daily basis can help to increase the numbers of good bacteria. Fermented foods (such as kefir) contain high levels of probiotics. The process of fermentation is one of the oldest existing ways to preserve foods, and it vastly increases the numbers of beneficial bacteria within them. It can be used to transform foods; for example, cabbage into sauerkraut, and milk into yoghurt and cheese. Fermentation is a common practice among most cultures. The Ancient Egyptians were the first to make yoghurt, which was the spontaneous result of camel milk being left out in the sweltering Northern African heat. Whereas over 4,000 years ago, cucumbers were pickled in the Middle East, in China fermented tea leaves gave rise to kombucha in around 200BCE. My personal favourite is kimchi (spicy pickled cabbage) and I am very fortunate that my sister-in-law, who originates from South Korea, is an expert at making it!

The process of fermentation relies on bacteria or yeasts that change the flavour and consistency of the food itself. At first glance this doesn't sound that appetising, but these foods have a unique taste and depth of flavour that add so much to enliven a meal. When looking for fermented foods, search for ones that contain live bacteria. Recent research from Stanford University published in the journal, *Cell*, showed that a 10-week course of a fibre- and fermented-food-rich diet, containing foods such as yoghurt, kefir, kimchi and kombucha, increased microbial diversity, which was enhanced by larger servings. Incredibly, results also showed that the levels of nineteen inflammatory markers were reduced in the blood as a result.[11] This small study reinforces the notion that we have the power to positively influence our GM, which in turn reduces inflammation.

Although there are no specific recommendations on a daily intake for probiotic foods, I would recommend trying to include at least one a day in your diet. Here's a list of probiotic foods to help you on your way:

Kimchi
Kombucha
Live yoghurt or kefir
Miso
Olives cured in water or brine
Pickles
Sauerkraut
Tempeh

Try fasting

In Chapter 4 we will take a deep dive into why fasting has benefits for our health; some of the things it can potentially help with
include blood pressure, weight management and heart health.
Fasting also helps the good bacteria to flourish, as friendly species such as *Akkermansia muciniphila* and *Bacteroides fragilis*
can survive periods without food, whereas bad bacteria are less
resilient and die.

There are many different ways to fast, but the one I often discuss with my patients is to try eating within a time window, also
known as intermittent fasting (see Chapter 4). Early evidence has
shown that fasting can improve microbial diversity and increased
production of anti-inflammatory SCFA compounds (explained
on page 89).[12] It seems as though aligning our mealtimes within
a specified time also helps to align digestion with our internal
body clock, known as our circadian rhythm. It's important to
note that intermittent fasting isn't for everyone, and it is not
suitable if you have a history of disordered or restrictive eating,
or you are taking certain medications.

Food for thought

We are riding the wave of a gut-health revolution. We know
more now about the profound and fascinating role that our gut
microbes play in our overall health and well-being than ever
before. From our brain to our skin, the trillions of bugs living in
the lining of our gut are orchestrating our immune system, our
hormones and how we think and feel. We have the extraordinary

power to support our gut microbiome, improve diversity and restore balance simply by paying attention to what we eat, so my only question now is: what are you waiting for?

Key skin-friendly takeaways

1. Our gut and skin are closely connected.

2. Imbalances in our gut microbiome can increase overall inflammation that impacts our skin.

3. Our diet holds the key to improving the gut microbiome and reducing inflammation.

4. Focus on increasing the variety of plants in your diet to support good bacteria and overall gut health.

5. Incorporate prebiotic and probiotic foods into your diet to improve the diversity of your gut microbes.

4

The SkinFood Approach

Nutrition is how we take care of our skin from the inside out. As we have learnt, many skincare products and creams simply can't reach the deeper layers of the skin, which is why we must turn to what's on our plate instead. Nutrients in the food we eat provide our skin with the building blocks it needs to be healthy, and they can have a huge impact on the overall appearance of our skin. We've already covered some of the foods and supplements that it might be helpful to incorporate into your diet, but the question of how to overhaul your approach to food might still feel quite daunting.

To make things as straightforward as possible, I've devised the SkinFood approach, which puts skin health at the top of the agenda. Devised from years of research and working with patients, it's easy, simple and, most importantly, flexible. It is not a diet or a quick fix, but rather a framework that can be adapted to fit your lifestyle, cultural preferences and food choices, because everyone has different budgets and needs. Think of this approach as the basis for overall happier, healthier skin that can also be adapted to address a specific skin concern, such as acne or ageing well – although it will take around 2–4 weeks to notice an improvement (the next chapter will offer tailored nutritional advice for the most common complaints I see in the clinic with guidance on how it can be implemented).

I am a passionate cook, and I love sharing meals with friends and family. Food is so much more than just nutrients. Eating is such a pleasurable experience, connecting us to the people around us, our heritage and even our travels. The smell of frying onions, garlic and ginger immediately transports me back to childhood, peeling garlic in the kitchen for my granny while she cooked dhal, chicken curry and rice. Grilling fish on the barbeque brings back nostalgic memories of holidays in Crete when my children were tiny. If we attempt to dissociate food from the important part it plays in the tapestry of our lives, and see it just as a necessity, we are depriving ourselves of one of life's greatest enjoyments.

I don't believe in cutting out whole food groups, so with this approach there is also always room for sweet treats, alcohol or any other indulgence – the key is balance and moderation. If a nutritious diet forms the foundation of what you eat, you should never feel guilty for enjoying a slice of cake or a bowl of ice cream. But all too often, I come across questionable advice for very restrictive eating plans, cutting out all gluten, dairy, sugar, and more, in an attempt to clear skin conditions. Although I do believe that certain foods may need to be eliminated from your diet if you have a genuine allergy or intolerance, cutting out multiple food groups is not a cure-all for treating skin conditions. (I will be discussing food allergies in Chapter 6.)

Many of my patients have embarked on extreme detoxes or 'cleanses' in an attempt to soothe their skin before coming to see me. Our body does not need to go on a detox: our liver and kidneys are designed to do just that. It is also important to remember that adopting an extreme approach to food is not sustainable. Sometimes a skin condition may appear to improve, but this may be temporary with the same condition rearing its head again only a few months down the line, leading to frustration and disappointment. You deserve to eat and enjoy the foods that you love, and to care for your skin – and the important thing to remember is that it's absolutely possible to do both.

The evolution of the SkinFood approach

Over the years I have met countless patients who have tried every type of diet imaginable: gluten-free, dairy-free, Paleo, Atkins, keto, Pagano – you name it. After listening to their stories, I knew that a popular diet approach to skin wasn't the answer, and it became my mission to come up with something targeted to skin health that was sustainable and enjoyable. It seemed that I'd assigned myself a near-impossible task.

From my research I understood how closely our skin and health are connected, and this led me to put my scientist hat on and spend many hours obsessively reading scientific papers in order to find out which foods and nutrients would not only support skin health but our overall well-being too. Hundreds of research papers later, I had come up with the SkinFood approach, which is founded on four key principles:

1 Eat to **GLOW:**
   Greens
   Lean proteins
   Oils and healthy fats
   Whole grains
2 Eat prebiotic and probiotic foods daily to support gut health.

3 Include anti-inflammatory spices, such as turmeric and cinnamon, in your meals.
4 Moderate your alcohol and refined sugar intake.

Why it works

The SkinFood approach is, at its essence, an anti-inflammatory way of eating, because inflammation lies at the heart of every skin concern, from eczema to premature skin ageing. Beyond the skin, inflammation also contributes to many other health conditions, including heart disease, and even certain cancers.

Some foods help to reduce inflammation because of the powerful compounds they contain, such as antioxidants and omega-3 fats, whereas foods such as white starch, processed meats (such as sausages and hams) and saturated fats can contribute to inflammation. We think this is why what is known as a Western diet – a diet high in refined starches, sugars and animal products – is linked to increased long-term health conditions such as type-2 diabetes and also certain skin concerns such as acne and psoriasis.

What then should we be eating instead? Well, imagine that you're sitting in a beachside taverna on a remote Greek island, enjoying a simple lunch of ripe tomato salad, freshly grilled fish with a squeeze of lemon and warm bread, all doused in fragrant olive oil. Sounds delicious? It is, and it might just be one of the healthiest ways we can eat.

The archetypal diet of countries such as Greece, Italy and Spain is known as the Mediterranean diet. It first rose to prominence in the seventies when a group of researchers, led by physiologist Dr Ancel Keys, sought to investigate the eating habits of people from across the world to explore why some lived longer than others. The Seven Countries Study compared the diets with disease rates in countries across the globe including the USA, Italy, Greece and Japan.[1] This pioneering study provided the first insight into how to eat for a long and healthy life. Researchers found that people living in countries like Italy and Greece had lower risks of heart disease and other medical conditions, and thus lived longer healthier lives. In fact, Dr Keys put his own research into practice, living until the age of 100 and remaining active in research until ninety-seven!

Decades later, the Mediterranean diet still comes out on top in studies on the healthiest way to eat. More recently, a group of researchers from the National Geographic, led by Dan Beuttner, studied the inhabitants of areas of the world where people live longest. They named these locations 'the Blue Zones', and one place that stood out was the Greek island of Ikaria, where people seemed to live to a much older age; in fact, it was not uncommon to live to 100. This phenomenon even became the basis of a *New York Times* magazine article entitled 'The island where people forget to die'.

It is believed that the simple approach to food in Ikaria, as well as other Mediterranean countries, is what holds the secret to longevity. The traditional diet on the island consisted largely of fruit, vegetables, pulses (including beans and lentils) and plenty of olive oil and oily fish, with little in the way of processed foods, red meat or refined sugar; however, red wine was enjoyed regularly. In addition to diet, a more relaxed way of life with greater social interaction and movement is also thought to contribute to the Ikarians' extraordinary lifespan. Although many countries around the Mediterranean have slightly different diets, it is this traditional Greek diet that we refer to as the 'Mediterranean diet'.

Still unconvinced? Here are just some of the benefits the Mediterranean diet boasts:

- Reduces the incidence of heart attacks, strokes and death from heart disease.
- Lowers the rates of developing certain types of cancer.
- Reduces the occurrence of Alzheimer's dementia.
- Lowers the likelihood of developing type-2 diabetes.
- Benefits weight management.
- Improves the gut microbiome and its proportion of good bacteria.
- Helps symptoms of depression.
- Increases telomere length (which as we know is linked to healthy ageing!).
- Positively impacts the skin.
- Lowers the risk of skin cancer reported (observed in a study of over 90,000 French women who followed a Mediterranean diet).[2]
- Reduced severity of psoriasis linked to eating a Mediterranean diet in a study of 150,000 French participants.[3]
- Less severe acne in a study of 51 people and lower levels of IGF-1, a key hormone linked to acne.[4]

Although there are clearly many proven health benefits derived from following a Mediterranean diet, this approach to food hasn't yet been optimised for skin health, which means it inevitably doesn't fulfil all the needs of my patients. Therefore, in order to create a truly inclusive, 360-degree plan for nourished skin, I decided to draw on the principles of the Mediterranean diet but to adapt them into my unique SkinFood approach. Here are some of the fundamental differences that I encourage.

- At the risk of sounding like a broken record, the relationship between the gut and the skin is hugely important, so any skin-friendly diet needs to promote a healthy gut microbiome. An effective way to do this is through the daily inclusion of probiotic and prebiotic foods.
- Although red wine is a prominent part of the Mediterranean diet, I am much more cautious about recommending it when it comes to skin health. Not only can alcohol cause flare-ups for many skin concerns, such as psoriasis and rosacea, but it can also accelerate skin ageing.
- Nuts, seeds and other healthy fats should be eaten daily, as they provide good sources of polyunsaturated fats and omega-3 that are critical for skin health. These fats moisturise the skin from within, support the skin barrier and help to calm inflammation.
- I also recommend incorporating anti-inflammatory spices such as turmeric into your diet. Spices with anti-inflammatory properties have been studied in depth in recent years, and although they don't feature in the Mediterranean diet, they have been used in Eastern cultures for centuries to benefit skin health.

GLOW on your plate – how to put it all together

A balanced plate is at the core of the SkinFood approach, as it helps to keep your blood sugar stable, while improving your energy levels and allowing room for nutrient-dense foods to meet your skin's needs.

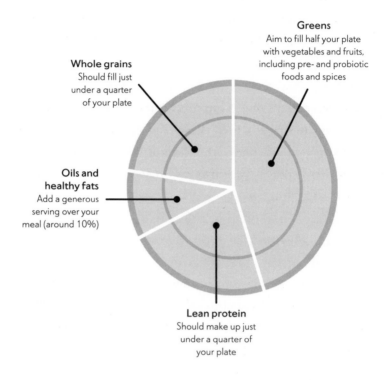

Greens
Aim to fill half your plate with vegetables and fruits, including pre- and probiotic foods and spices

Whole grains
Should fill just under a quarter of your plate

Oils and healthy fats
Add a generous serving over your meal (around 10%)

Lean protein
Should make up just under a quarter of your plate

The GLOW plate: a visual example of the quantities to eat in a typical meal.

The diagram above is an example of what a typical plate of food might look like (but see below for more about portion sizes). Here is what to aim for:

- About half your plate comprising fresh vegetables/ fruits with some pre- and probiotic foods and spices.
- Equal amounts of whole grains and lean protein

(plant-based protein works nicely too). If you want
to include some dairy products such as cheese or
yoghurt, go ahead.

- Don't skimp on skin-loving healthy fats; these can be
from healthy oils, as well as nuts and seeds, which
contain nutrients and vitamins.

Remember, not all meals have to look like this, mine certainly
don't, but this is what we want to aim for throughout the
day. When we think about how we nourish our body, it is
the long-term patterns rather than individual plates of food
that matter.

Portion sizes

I'm not overly prescriptive about portion sizes. It really does
depend on your individual level of activity, age and other factors, but if you would like an approximate rule of thumb, the
following is a sensible guide for a typical meal:

- Two handfuls of fresh fruit and vegetables – aim
for seven portions per day (each handful is roughly
one portion).
- One palm-sized portion of protein – aim for two
portions per day.
- One palm-sized portion of whole grains – aim for three
portions per day.
- A generous helping of healthy fats such as a tablespoon
of nuts or oil – aim for two tablespoons of olive oil and
one small handful of nuts or seeds per day.

In Chapter 10, you'll find delicious, quick and easy recipes that reflect the principles of the GLOW plate; however, if you're raring to go and looking for inspiration, here are some examples of easy meals and snacks that you might want to try making:

- Roasted vegetables cooked in olive oil with a hummus and feta wholegrain wrap.
- Egg and avocado topped with seeds on wholegrain toast.
- Wholemeal pizza topped with tomato, veggies and cheese, and a side salad dressed with olive oil and nuts.
- Live yoghurt with fruits and seedy wholegrain granola.

When planning your meals, remember that food doesn't fall neatly into categories; for example, an avocado is a fruit, a source of healthy fats, and naturally high in fibre too. Here's a nutritional breakdown to help you visualise (values are per 100g avocado):

6.7g fibre
2.7g protein
14.7g fat (mainly monounsaturated)
Minerals: copper, potassium, zinc and magnesium
Vitamins: B5, B9, E and C

In terms of how you spread your meals out, it is a matter of personal preference. In general, three meals per day and two snacks helps you to feel full, satisfied and nourished, but, as always, this can be adapted to your lifestyle. We'll now move on to breaking down the GLOW plate, so that we can understand the role each component plays in helping to promote healthy skin.

Eat your greens ... and every other colour too

Fruit and vegetables are some of our richest sources of antioxidants, which is why they are a vital element of the SkinFood approach. These extraordinary compounds fight ageing and skin inflammation at a deeper level than skincare products alone can reach.

Not only do plants provide us with a multitude of vitamins, minerals and powerful anti-inflammatory compounds, they also contain high amounts of fibre, which, as we have learned, feed good gut bacteria. Importantly, fruit and vegetables also add a delicious flavour and texture to meals, and although we hear so much about 'eating your five a day', I really believe that we should be aiming for closer to seven a day.

When it comes to planning meals with fruits and vegetables, try to be adventurous and incorporate as varied a mix of plants as possible. One way to increase our variety is to think about colour. You might have come across the phrase 'eat the rainbow' before and found it gimmicky, but there is genuine science behind it. The compounds found in fruit and vegetables that give them their unique colour also have incredible antioxidant effects, as we can see in the table below:

Red	Tomatoes contain lycopene, and levels increase as it is cooked. This antioxidant has been shown to protect the skin against harmful UV light
Orange	Beta carotene in carrots, sweet potatoes and peppers is both anti-inflammatory and antioxidant

Yellow	Peaches, yellow peppers and pineapples contain bioflavonoids. These help to boost vitamin C, which targets wrinkles and age spots
Green	Spinach, broccoli and kale are among the best sources of lutein, an antioxidant shown to protect skin from UV damage
Blue	Blueberries, blackberries and dark grapes all contain a variety of phytochemicals, including anthocyanins, which give them their rich colour. Their anti-inflammatory effects deter collagen breakdown and fight premature ageing
Purple	Beetroot and purple potato contain betalains, another exceptionally potent antioxidant, which quenches inflammation

The antioxidant qualities in differently coloured
fruits and vegetables.

You can make easy steps towards increasing how many plants you eat by trying to include more fruits and vegetables at mealtimes, starting with a handful of berries at breakfast, a plum and some nuts as a snack, tomato salad and a wholegrain sandwich at lunch, and a vegetable and chickpea curry with bulgur wheat for dinner.

Don't feel that you have to be limited to fresh fruit and vegetables, as they can be costly. Why not try dried fruit instead? A small handful of around 30g makes up one portion and works perfectly as a quick and tasty snack, but be mindful not to have more than one portion per day, as too much can lead to spikes in blood sugar. Frozen fruit and vegetables are another simple and economical way to improve the variety in your diet. They retain all of the nutritional benefit of their fresh counterparts and there is less waste, as they can be stashed in the freezer for whenever you need them. Frozen berries, mangoes, mixed vegetables, peas, beans, spinach, butternut squash, cabbage and more can be quickly used to make smoothies, soups and curries.

Lean protein

Protein forms the building blocks of our entire body, from the skin, hair and nails to the muscles and organs. Proteins are made up of individual amino acids that are broken down in the gut and absorbed into the bloodstream, and they then travel to where they are needed for tissue regeneration and repair. Of these twenty-two amino acids, eight are essential and must be consumed in our diet as our body cannot make them by itself, as we discussed in Chapter 2.

How much protein is right for you will depend on several factors, such as your age or whether you have increased requirements (for example pregnancy or recent recovery from an illness), so remember to adapt your meals accordingly to make sure that they're tailored to suit your needs. As a rule of thumb, most adults require a minimum of 0.75g of protein per kilo of body weight (for example, a 60kg woman would need 45g of protein each day).

Complete proteins contain all the required essential amino acids and include fish, eggs, soya, meat and dairy. There's a common misconception that you can't get adequate protein from a vegan or vegetarian diet, and although most individual vegetarian protein sources do not contain all eight essential amino acids, combining different foods helps to meet our nutritional requirements. We should all be trying to eat more plant-based sources of protein, both for our own health and for that of the environment. Vegetarian protein sources also come with added benefits such as fibre and vitamins. In the table below I've outlined how different protein sources match up for comparison:

Food type	Protein content g/100g
Chicken breast	32
Tuna (tinned)	24.9
Salmon	24.6
Cod	23.9
Almonds	21.1
Walnuts	14.1
Egg (whole)	14
Wheat flour (brown)	12.2
Cooked chickpeas	9.5
Cottage cheese	9.4
Tofu	8.1
Red lentils (boiled)	7.6
Plain Greek-style yoghurt	5.7

The protein content of different foods.

Many foods, including nuts and seeds, whole grains and even vegetables, contain high levels of protein, so you don't necessarily need protein supplements to meet your daily requirements unless you are exercising heavily.

If you've tended to focus on meat as your main source of protein, try experimenting with tofu and pulses as an alternative. Oily fish is also a good option, as it has wonderful health benefits, as we have seen: it's rich in omega-3 and astaxanthin, and they work together to protect skin moisture and scavenge free radicals. As part of a Mediterranean approach to food, fish is recommended twice or three times per week, with current recommendations suggesting that two of these portions should be oily fish. We often veer towards salmon when choosing oily fish, but there are other options including mackerel, trout and sardines. Both fresh and tinned are good choices, but if you prefer to go with tinned, which is generally more economical, I'd recommend looking for options that have been preserved in spring water.

One thing to always be mindful of when shopping is that our choices have wider implications on the planet, so when it comes to fish I would recommend going with sustainably sourced options where possible. Sustainable fish are caught or produced in a way that enables stocks to replenish without causing unnecessary damage to marine life (you can find more information at www.mcsuk.org).

Oils and healthy fats

Healthy oils, nuts, seeds and oily fish are rich in polyunsaturated fats (including omega-3), which have important anti-inflammatory effects on the skin. When we don't eat enough of these good fats, our skin can end up appearing dry and dull. I'm a huge fan of healthy fats, as they offer so many benefits for the skin and beyond, including stabilising blood sugar and helping to keep you feeling satisfied and full, so I recommend incorporating them into meals wherever possible.

Studies have shown that omega-3 fatty acids can also reduce inflammation in acne lesions, help to prevent dry eyes in rosacea, reduce the severity of psoriasis and support healthy ageing too. And, of course, as we've already learnt, healthy fats are essential in maintaining our skin barrier and helping to keep it supple and hydrated.

Here are my top choices for healthy oils. Try to look for cold-pressed where possible, as cold-pressed oils generally have higher levels of nutrients and are less processed:

Olive oil	Rich in anti-inflammatory oleic acid and skin-loving vitamin E. When using for cooking make sure not to overheat until smoking, as this causes changes in the fat content, making it less healthy
Walnut oil	Great for salad dressings (not for cooking), as it contains high levels of omega-3
Avocado oil	Great for salads, dips or baking. It is high in both monounsaturated fatty acids and antioxidants
Flaxseed oil	This particular oil is perfect for salad dressings. I don't recommend cooking with it, as it smokes at a low temperature. It is the oil richest in omega-3
Rapeseed oil	This affordable oil is naturally high in unsaturated fat including omega-3

The benefits of healthy oils explained.

You might have come across recipes and articles online promoting the use of coconut oil and its health benefits and wonder why it's not included in this list. Coconut oil contains 80–90 per cent saturated fat, although around 50 per cent of this is a type called medium-chain triglycerides, which are marginally more beneficial. Because of its saturated fat content, it can raise levels of bad cholesterol, so I am cautious when recommending it and would advise minimising your intake if you have a history of heart disease or high cholesterol. Use it for flavour and authenticity in recipes such as curries, but when it comes to general daily use,

I would suggest sticking to one of the healthier options I have mentioned in the table above.

Nuts and seeds

I recommend eating a small handful of nuts and seeds every day if you can. They are nutrient powerhouses packed with good fats, vitamins, minerals and proteins. To make sure I'm incorporating them into my diet, every evening I prepare a snack box filled with nuts and berries that I pop in my bag the next morning so that I have something to take with me to work. It's an easy snack that needs almost no preparation, plus it's satisfying (more on this in Chapter 10). If you are allergic to a specific nut or seed, don't worry, there are plenty of alternative sources, including the oils mentioned above, avocados, oily fish or, if necessary, an omega-3 supplement is also worth considering.

This table acts as a simple guide to the health benefits of different varieties of nuts and seeds:

Walnuts	Walnuts contain the highest levels of omega-3 and antioxidants of any nut, which makes them my go-to snack.
Almonds	Raw, roasted or whizzed into a butter, almonds contain vitamin E, protein and help good bacteria such as *Bifidobacteria* and *Lactobacillus* to thrive.
Cashew nuts	Cashews contain healthy fats, protein, vitamin K and magnesium. They also contain zinc and copper.
Brazil nuts	Brazil nuts are packed with omega-3 and selenium, but be careful not to overdo it (no more than one per day).

Flaxseeds	Flaxseeds contain a type of antioxidant called lignans at higher levels than any other plant food. They are also fibre rich. Ground flaxseeds are more easily absorbed.
Pumpkin seeds	Pumpkin seeds contain zinc in addition to healthy fats. Low zinc levels can be linked to dry skin and breakouts.
Sunflower seeds	Sunflower seeds are abundant in vitamins B and E, as well as selenium.
Hemp seeds	Hemp seeds are high in selenium and omega-3 and are also a good source of protein.
Chia seeds	Chia seeds contain high levels of plant-based omega-3.

The health benefits of nuts and seeds.

Whole grains

In recent years carbohydrates have been demonised as the root of many health problems, but they actually form an integral part of our diet. Whole grains are high in carbohydrates and come with many benefits; for example, they are a rich source of fibre, which helps to feed our good gut bacteria and keeps us feeling fuller for longer, stabilising our blood sugar. The key to enjoying carbohydrates is to choose the right ones and to eat them in suitable amounts. Refined carbohydrates, such as white bread, pastries, many breakfast cereals and white rice, offer fewer nutritional benefits due to the way in which they have been processed, but they are not inherently 'bad foods'.

We learned about the glycaemic index on page 60, and it gives us some idea of how our blood sugar levels respond to the food we eat. Although this isn't a perfect science, and different people can react differently to the same foods, it does help to inform us about the foods that have a lower and more stabilising effect on blood sugar, including many whole grains. Foods that are more likely to cause blood sugar spikes (such as sweets, biscuits and white carbohydrates) are more likely to contribute to cravings and energy slumps. Keeping blood sugar stable is as much about feeling good as it is about looking good. As we discuss in the next chapter, high-glycaemic diets can trigger breakouts and accelerate skin ageing.

Your gut needs 30g of fibre a day to work well, so whole grains are a great way to help you reach that target, and they also offer the extra benefits of containing B vitamins and minerals, as well as protein. Aim for around three portions of whole grains per day, with each portion measuring approximately one handful or a medium slice of bread. In terms of choosing whole grains for your meals, look for foods such as:

Brown or wild rice
Bulgur wheat
Wholegrain oats
Quinoa
Spelt wheat
Wholegrain or multigrain bread (including wholegrain sourdough)
Wholegrain pasta
Wholegrain barley

NOTE Look specifically for 'wholegrain' on the food labels of your favourite foods, as the wholegrain option will carry more fibre, nutrients and vitamins. When it comes to wholegrain bread, a soya and linseed option has the added benefit of omega-3 fats and has a lower impact on blood sugar.

If you're feeling adventurous and want to change things up, here are some more unusual options to try:

Buckwheat
Kamut
Millet
Rye
Teff

Gluten and the skin

Gluten is a protein found in wheat, rye and barley, and I'm often asked if a gluten-free diet will benefit the skin. I am not a fan of cutting out gluten unless there is a legitimate reason, as doing so won't be a magic bullet for the skin. Although, as we'll learn in the following chapter, there are some specific instances where it can be helpful to omit gluten from the diet, for most people this is not the case. Remember that some gluten-free equivalents can have fewer vitamins than fortified foods containing gluten, while also including more highly processed ingredients and coming with a higher price tag.

Prebiotic and probiotic foods

Try to include prebiotic and probiotic foods in your meals at least once per day to help support your good gut bacteria. As we covered the health benefits of these foods in Chapter 3, I won't go into too much detail here, but the following list offers a quick reference guide to the foods that fall into either of these categories:

Prebiotic foods:

Garlic
Jerusalem artichoke
Leek
Legumes such as chickpeas and lentils
Onion
Whole grains

Probiotic foods:

Kefir
Kimchi
Kombucha
Live yoghurt
Miso
Sauerkraut

The sweet spot

You'll be glad to hear that sugar is *on* the menu as part of the SkinFood approach, although it's sensible to be mindful of the amount of refined or added sugars we consume. Remember that sugar encompasses everything from natural sugars found in fruits to refined white table sugar. When consumed in excess, sugar can lead to a myriad of health problems that are on the rise in the Western world, particularly type-2 diabetes and other long-term health concerns but it can also worsen certain skin conditions and accelerate skin ageing. Our current NHS guidelines advise no more than six teaspoons (30g) of sugar per day, which includes:

- Sugars in drinks (including fizzy drinks, sweetened juice and coffee).
- Sugars added to food (including flavoured yoghurt, cakes, biscuits, ready-made meals and sauces).
- Sugars found naturally in honey and syrups (maple, agave, coconut sugar/nectar and date nectar).

Be aware that food labels can be misleading. When you look at the ingredients breakdown, keep your eyes peeled for 'carbohydrates, of which sugars', as the given number will indicate how much sugar is in the food you are eating. Added sugars must also be listed in the ingredients, so keep an eye out for those too. You may be surprised to learn the sugar contents of some popular foods and drinks:

Starbucks caramel frappuccino (grande), 55g
Can of cola (330ml), 35g
Nature Valley oats and honey granola bars (1 serving), 11 g
Müllerlight strawberry yoghurt (175g serving), 12.4g
Aperol spritz (cocktail), 19g
Lipton peach iced tea (500ml), 22g

Unrefined sugars, such as maple syrup and coconut sugar, are often thought to be healthier options, but although they might have slightly more nutrients, our body still recognises them as sugar, and as such they still cause sharp rises in blood sugar levels. They also contain similar amounts of calories to table sugar.

Sugar is a part of life, we certainly don't have to fear it, but we do need to be mindful of how much we are consuming overall. One way to modulate the impact of sweet treats on blood sugar is to combine them with fat and fibre; for example, enjoying a dessert at the end of a meal rather than having a chocolate bar on its own. Other options to satisfy sweet cravings include:

- Chocolate-covered nuts and an apple.
- Chocolate, Banana and Buckwheat Loaf (page 343).
- The APPLE Study Muffins (page 340).
- Oatcake spread with nut butter and a little honey.
- Dates stuffed with ricotta and walnuts.

Choosing chocolate

As well as tasting silky and sweet, chocolate is rich in antioxidants such as catechins, anthocyanidins and proanthocyanidins. Chocolate is produced from cacao powder, which is usually combined with cocoa butter and sugar, but not all chocolate is created equal. Here are some tips to choosing nutritious (and delicious) options:

- Check the ingredients list to look for as few ingredients as possible: cocoa mass, sugar, cocoa butter and sometimes vanilla.

- Look for dark chocolate with at least 70 per cent cocoa, as higher percentages have greater concentrations of antioxidants.
- Good-quality dark chocolate should not have added milk.
- Choose Fairtrade when you can, as this helps to support farmers who grow and harvest cacao.
- Look for brands with a lower sugar content (for example about 30g sugar/100g chocolate).
- Despite its high sugar content, dark chocolate has a glycaemic index of 23 (low) because the fat it contains slows the absorption of sugar.
- Eating chocolate releases feel-good hormones such as dopamine, serotonin and oxytocin. Relax and enjoy!
- Be mindful of portion sizes and enjoy slowly to fully savour the flavour. A couple of squares (20g) of dark chocolate a day is fine by me.

The benefits of spices

In several cultures, including my own, spices are included in every meal of the day, from breakfast to dinner. Known to add incredible fragrance and flavour to meals, they also have important health benefits.

Turmeric

The golden spice, turmeric is commonly used in South-East Asian cooking. In Ayurvedic tradition it has long been used for its anti-inflammatory effects, and as a child in Sri Lanka I would have turmeric paste applied to any cuts or scrapes.

The active compound within turmeric is curcumin, and there has been extensive research carried out to understand its medicinal properties. Studies have shown that it is both an antioxidant and an anti-inflammatory and can even help in conditions such as arthritis. As yet we don't know if turmeric can clear skin conditions, but early research shows that it can reduce overall inflammation levels in the body.[5] I recommend trying to work turmeric into your diet, rather than taking it in the form of supplements. Its absorption and activity are improved when combined with a little black pepper.

If you're unfamiliar with turmeric but would like to find ways to incorporate it into your diet, why not try:

- Golden Sunshine Smoothie (page 299).
- Turmeric Roasted Chicken Salad (page 311).
- Adding it to curries and stews.
- Adding it to smoothies.

Cinnamon

I admit that I am biased when it comes to this lovely warming spice. Pure Ceylon cinnamon hails from my homeland, and this variety is thought to be the most superior in terms of both flavour and health benefits. Research has shown that just half a teaspoon of cinnamon per day can help to curb high blood sugar levels in those with type-2 diabetes, pre-diabetes or polycystic ovarian syndrome (PCOS),[6] a common hormonal imbalance in women that can provoke acne. Cinnamon is also packed with antioxidant compounds that our skin loves. You don't need a lot, and I wouldn't recommend taking it as a supplement, as too much of it can cause side effects and even harm the liver. Here are some simple ways to introduce cinnamon into your meals:

- Add it to your morning tea or coffee (Try my BeauTea Chai on page 292).
- Sprinkle it onto breakfast cereal, oats or yoghurt in the morning.
- Use it in your baking (I find it works especially well in cookies and banana bread).
- Add it to curries or stews.

(Cinnamon may occasionally cause flare-ups of pre-existing rosacea, so trial a small amount in the first instance.)

It's not just what you eat but *when* you eat

I am fascinated by the concept of intermittent fasting (IF) and its potential benefits for the skin. So much so that in fact it is part of our ongoing research project into the effect of diet on psoriasis at King's College London.

Intermittent fasting or 'time-restricted eating' is a more recent trend to surface that relies on principal meals being eaten within specific windows of time; for example, daily meals are eaten within an 8-hour period during the day (for example, between 12pm and 8pm) and you fast for the remaining 16 hours of the day. There are many different ways to fast, with some people choosing to reduce their calories for 2 days of the week, popularly known as the 5:2 diet.

Although it might seem new, it's a practice that has been

around for thousands of years and a customary part of many religions; for example, during Ramadan, Yom Kippur and Hindu religious ceremonies, people will fast for several hours. Recent scientific research, however, has brought to light many ways in which fasting could be good for our health.[7]

When we refrain from eating for about 12 hours, our body switches from using carbohydrates (glucose) for energy and starts to use our fat stores. These fats are broken down to release compounds called ketones. Ketones aren't just used for energy; they have numerous different effects on the body, including reducing inflammation and promoting tissue repair. Studies have shown that IF might also help with weight management, type-2 diabetes and lowering high cholesterol, and there is currently interest into whether it could be helpful in treating several inflammatory conditions such as arthritis as a complement to mainstream medical treatments.

Fasting for periods of time also helps to support the gut microbiome, encouraging good bacteria to grow while starving bad bacteria. Another benefit of intermittent fasting is that you tend to eat less late at night, and this is beneficial because eating a large, late meal has been shown to have adverse effects on blood sugar, causing it to stay raised for longer. It's thought that IF's stabilising effect on blood sugar might be partly responsible for its benefits.

The link between intermittent fasting and skin health is still being investigated, and the research project that I'm part of will go some way towards better understanding its effects; however, the anti-inflammatory benefits of fasting, combined with favourable impact on the gut microbiome and blood sugar certainly make it something worth considering for skin health.

Intermittent fasting in practice

How do you start? You can try bringing your evening meal forward by 1 hour and moving breakfast back by 1 hour, or you can eat within a 12-hour window (instead of an 8-hour window), say from 8am to 8pm, but make sure to drink water or other unsweetened drinks so that you stay hydrated during the fasting hours. Gradually, you will see that if you can shorten your eating window, say by an hour every few weeks, by the end you will have an 8-hour eating window. See how you go and whether it suits you – fasting doesn't suit everyone. From my experience in the clinic, some people find it to be helpful for weight management, and for improving energy levels and sleep quality, but I do not recommend it without the supervision of your healthcare provider or registered dietitian if you have a history of restrictive eating habits or disordered eating.

You are what you drink

What you drink is arguably just as important as what you eat. As you can see from the list on page 126, fizzy drinks, store-bought juices, energy drinks and some syrup-sweetened coffees can be high in refined sugar, with some immediately exceeding your recommended daily intake of sugar!

Alcohol, as I have mentioned, doesn't cause problems for everyone, but if you have eczema, psoriasis or rosacea it can be an issue. There is also research that has shown that drinking more than eight alcoholic drinks per week accelerates facial ageing. Pass the water please!

Tea and coffee often have a bad reputation when it comes

to skin, but they actually contain antioxidants called polyphe-nols. Although coffee boasts more antioxidants than tea, it also contains roughly twice the amount of caffeine. For adults, the general advice is not to exceed 400µg per day, and the table below can help you gauge how much you're having. Too much caffeine can lead to heart palpitations, high blood pressure and anxiety – and also drive the stress hormone cortisol, reduce blood flow to the skin and cause dehydration that leaves the skin dull and dry.

Green tea is a wonderful alternative to tea and coffee that contains even more potent antioxidants. It is made from the same plant as black tea but it isn't processed to the same degree. It is thought that this is why it is so rich in a type of antioxidant called catechin or epigallocatechin-3-gallate (EGCG). Matcha green tea is also gaining popularity and is said to contain even more antioxidants than conventional green tea. Matcha is grown slightly differently from other varieties and is prepared in its own unique way. Its leaves are stone ground to form a fine powder that is used to brew tea, which means that you end up consuming more of the leaf itself, and this affords around double the amount of catechins.

Green tea has been studied for a range of medical conditions including Alzheimer's and certain cancers too. Research also suggests it might help to prevent skin cancer and even stave off hair loss. After learning about the science, I now regularly drink green tea throughout the day after my morning coffee.

Beverage	Caffeine
Instant coffee	82µg
Matcha green tea	70µg

Tea (standard tea bag)	45µg
Espresso	27µg
Green tea	20µg
Decaf coffee	3µg

The caffeine content of teas and coffees in an average serving.

Hydration and your skin

We often hear that drinking eight glasses (or 2 litres) of water a day is the recipe for glowing skin, shrinking pores and plumping wrinkles. Our skin does need water, and when we are dehydrated, it loses elasticity and doesn't bounce back as it should. Making sure that we are properly hydrated also helps to support blood flow to the skin, which delivers nutrients and removes waste products, but science doesn't back up the recommendation to glug litres of water each day. One research study looked at the impact of drinking water on skin wrinkles and overall smoothness, and after four weeks of observation they noticed no difference in the participants' skin.[8] Although drinking water might not turn back the clock, you'll still feel better for it, however. Current guidance advises six to eight glasses of a fluid per day, and you may need more if you're exercising a lot or you live in a warm climate, so keep hydrated, and aim to drink enough so that your urine is pale yellow in colour.

Key skin-friendly takeaways

1. The SkinFood approach forms a flexible framework around which to build your meals.

2. Keep the balanced plate in mind when planning meals and think GLOW (greens, lean protein/plant-based protein, oils and whole grains).

3. There is always room for treats and the things you love – it is a matter of moderation.

4. Eat the rainbow: brightly coloured fruits and vegetables are excellent for skin health.

5. Include good fats at every meal, including healthy oils, nuts and seeds.

6. Chocolate is on the menu, but choose wisely.

7. Include prebiotic and probiotic foods in your daily diet to support gut health.

8. Pay attention to what you drink as well as what you eat.

5

Optimising Nutrition for Specific Skin Concerns

The experience I have gained from over a decade in dermatology, talking to thousands of people about their skin, has led me to develop the SkinFood approach. While the principles of the approach remain the same across the board, personalising it helps to address individual skin concerns. To develop this advice, I have drawn on both the latest rigorous scientific research as well as my own experiences from the clinic.

What you'll find in this chapter are answers to the most common questions that I'm asked by patients. My aim is to recreate a conversation that we might have were you to see me for a consultation so that I'm able to offer tailored nutritional advice for your skin. The recommendations are customised to address the most common skin concerns: acne, premature ageing and a loss of radiance, psoriasis and rosacea. A gentle reminder again that if your skin condition is not improving or it's affecting your mental health, please do make an appointment with your doctor for further treatment.

Nutrition for acne

Who hasn't experienced spots, zits, pimples or breakouts at some time or another? Acne is the single most common skin concern that I see in the clinic, and one that, fortunately, we can treat effectively by addressing triggers and optimising nutrition. Keep the foundation of the SkinFood approach in mind, and get ready to embark on an acne deep dive.

The acne–diet spectrum

A survey of people with acne found that over 90 per cent thought that food was an aggravating factor for their skin, and although it's easy to assume that acne is caused by a 'bad diet',[1] this is actually a common myth that needs debunking. Some of my acne patients are dietitians or nutritionists themselves, and they would not be coming to see me if food offered a universal fix. As we learned earlier, the reality is that not everyone responds to food in the same way.[2] Some people have tried detox cleanses and every type of diet imaginable to clear their skin without seeing any benefits, but for others simply reducing refined sugar can effectively clear breakouts. Rather than assuming that there's a straightforward relationship between diet and acne, I have come to understand that instead we should consider it a spectrum: what I refer to as the acne–diet spectrum.

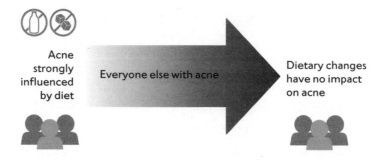

The acne–diet spectrum. For some people, acne is strongly influenced by diet, whereas for others diet does not seem to play much of a role. In the middle of this spectrum are those who may notice some changes in their acne with relation to their diet, but other factors such as hormones and stress can also contribute.

At one end of the spectrum, there are those whose breakouts are easily triggered by what they eat: for example, eat too much refined sugar, dairy or greasy foods and a spot will appear, quite literally, overnight. Simple changes to their diet make a huge difference in these instances. At the other end of the spectrum are people for whom excluding foods makes little or no difference to their breakouts. Instead, their acne is more strongly influenced by hormones, genetics, stress and other factors. The two patient cases from the clinic described in this chapter illustrate opposite ends of the acne–diet spectrum.

Which end of the acne–diet spectrum are you on? Maybe you fall somewhere in the middle, where dietary triggers can play a role, but so can hormones or stress. I've found that explaining the acne–diet spectrum to patients really helps to break the cycle of self-blame that can come with living with acne, and it provides a sense of relief that can have a positive influence on their relationship with food. Remember, as we learned in Skin School in Chapter 1, that even if your acne is strongly influenced by diet, food is not the *cause* but instead should be considered a *trigger*.

Wherever you fall on the acne–diet spectrum, the SkinFood approach will help you to feel good and should be the first step in your skincare routine, because, as we know, the approach is rich in anti-inflammatory healthy fats and vibrant, antioxidant-rich fruits and vegetables. These potent compounds can help to reduce inflammation and support skin healing after acne breakouts.

Which foods can trigger acne?

Research studies point to two main types of foods that can potentially trigger breakouts:

1. High glycaemic-index (GI) foods, including refined sugar (think biscuits, sweets, sweetened fizzy drinks, cakes, and so on).
2. Dairy products, particularly low-fat milk (see below).

Some people also think that greasy or fatty foods can make their breakouts worse, but the research in this area is a little weaker. The research in this field is still evolving and so far no single study has proven a direct link between food and acne, but the current findings suggest there could be some correlation. As such, a recent guide for doctors managing acne published by the UK's National Institute for Health and Care Excellence (NICE) did not specify dietary recommendations for acne, but instead emphasised the importance of maintaining a generally healthy diet. There are also concerns that dietary restrictions can lead to obsessive eating habits and disorders in people who are already vulnerable to low self-esteem. This is certainly something I have encountered in the clinic and why I never recommend restrictive diets.

The UK guidance, however, differs somewhat from our colleagues over the pond. In the US, the American Academy of Dermatologists acknowledge that there is some emerging evidence indicating high glycaemic-index foods and dairy products, particularly low-fat milk, can contribute to acne and I have therefore reflected these in the box above. Considering the evidence so far, my aim is to provide you with a balanced and sensible way to explore the role of diet in managing your acne.

A word of caution

Over the years, I have come across many people who have needlessly tried cutting out several food groups and even developed restrictive eating habits or eating disorders, in a desperate attempt to control their skin. They may even have undertaken food intolerance testing, which has no place in acne management at all (more on this in Chapter 6). If this sounds familiar to you, please see your doctor (you'll find further advice in the Resources section).

Simone's case study below gives an example of how such eating habits can creep up on us. Furthermore, don't let searching for dietary acne triggers delay you from seeking medical treatment. This is particularly important if you have scarring, you have cystic acne or your acne is affecting your mental health or quality of life. The 4-Step Skin Solution incorporates nutrition, skincare and medical treatment for those who need it; it isn't simply a case of one step will fix everything.

CASE STUDY: ACNE AND A RESTRICTIVE DIET

Simone was a university student when she first came to see me, and her acne had been on and off since she was a teenager. She had tried many treatments over the years including creams, facials and even laser, but her acne remained persistent. When she first walked into my office she was anxious and worried. She had inflamed sore pimples over her cheeks and chin and red marks that her acne had left behind too.

She told me that she had been on a detox cleanse for 2 months in an attempt to clear her skin, cutting out all dairy, gluten, sugar, coffee and alcohol. She was miserable. And the worst part was that her acne had barely improved. We talked about how much her skin had affected her and left her feeling embarrassed and unhappy, so I explained the acne–diet spectrum to her and emphasised that the stress of following such a rigid regime could even add to her emotional burden.

Instead, I suggested the following:

- **Step 1** Simone was advised to focus on incorporating the nutritional principles of the SkinFood approach, which doesn't require exclusion of any sort and is rich in antioxidants and proteins required for wound repair and scar healing. Simone immediately took to the plan because of its flexibility and focus on overall balance rather than restriction, which meant that she no longer had to spend time laboriously weighing food or thinking about all the things she wasn't allowed to eat.

- **Step 2** We introduced a daily mindfulness practice to help Simone manage stress.
- **Step 3** I recommended products so that Simone could create a reliable acne-clearing skincare routine.
- **Step 4** Finally, I suggested Simone use a prescription retinol cream at night and azelaic acid cream in the morning.

When she returned 8 weeks later, she was very pleased with the progress that her skin had made, but more importantly she felt much better in herself. She was able to enjoy meals again without constantly fearing breakouts.

I am fortunate to work alongside a team of experienced dietitians who specialise in helping people who have developed disordered or restrictive eating habits, so if you feel the above could apply to you, please seek help from a qualified professional.

Is sugar to blame for acne?

As we know, the Western diet is generally higher in refined sugar, and researchers have wondered whether this, along with increased amounts of dairy, starchy carbohydrates and saturated fats in typical Western meals, could explain rising rates of acne.

Several large studies, looking at thousands of participants have linked acne to high-glycaemic foods.[2] I described this on page 60, but here is a quick recap on the glycaemic index (GI). It's a scale used to refer to how quickly a given food can cause a rise in blood sugar. Here are some examples of high-GI foods:

Biscuits
Cakes
Flavoured syrups added to tea and coffee
Hidden sugars in breakfast cereals, condiments, drinks
Sugary soft drinks
Sweets
White sugar
White bread, bagels and baguettes

Looking at this list, you'll recognise that these are the foods we know we should be careful about eating in excess, not just to protect our skin but for our overall well-being. A high-sugar diet can be linked to other long-term health conditions, such as type-2 diabetes and heart disease. Mia's case below illustrates how, for some people, excess refined sugar can contribute to acne breakouts.

CASE STUDY: ACNE AND A HIGH-SUGAR DIET

Mia came to see me just after COVID lockdown. Like so many others, she had moved to working from home and spent long days in front of the computer alone in her flat. Her skin had slowly started to break out more often. In the past, she had experienced a couple of spots each month before her menstrual cycle, but in the last year these had become more frequent, with red painful spots on her cheeks and chin pretty much every day. She had researched skincare online and had tried several spot creams from the pharmacy, but still every few days, a new pimple would appear, so I asked Mia whether she'd made any changes to her lifestyle, including her diet. She revealed that she had felt bored and lonely working at her desk at home, and it wasn't uncommon for her to finish a couple of bags of sweets as she worked, with a can or two of fizzy drinks. This added up to around 70g of refined sugar per day, double the recommended upper limit. Here's how we managed Mia's acne using the 4-Step Skin Solution:

- **Step 1** We talked about easy steps to try to reduce refined sugar and the broader nutritional principles of the SkinFood approach. She swapped sweets for nutritious snacks such as berries and nuts and switched cola for sparkling water with slices of lemon and cucumber.
- **Step 2** We also thought that going for a daily walk would be a great way for her to take a break from her work, boost her mood and get some fresh air and exercise.
- **Step 3** Mia's skincare routine was good, so didn't require changing.
- **Step 4** I gave Mia a prescription for a retinol and benzoyl peroxide cream to help tackle her spots.

I saw Mia 8 weeks later and was impressed with her progress and pleased that most of her spots had cleared, but she had a surprise for me. Shortly after our appointment Mia had lost the prescription she had been given, so she decided to go with the dietary and lifestyle changes that we had discussed and her skin had started to clear. Not only that, but she also had more energy and felt better — exactly what having an even blood sugar level should feel like. For Mia, a diet high in refined sugars had triggered an acne flare, and changing what she ate made all the difference, not just to her skin but for her health too.

In 2020, a French research study looked at the diets of over 20,000 people and found that those who ate more milk chocolate, sweets and sugary drinks had a greater chance of experiencing acne.[4] Although such studies can suggest an association, they don't definitively prove that there is a link. In order to establish this, further studies, including clinical trials, need to be carried out, and so far a total of six trials have looked at the effect of a lower GI diet on acne. In these trials, participants with acne are divided into two groups: one group follows a low-GI diet, reducing the amounts of refined-sugar foods, while the other group follows a standard diet.

Out of the six trials that have taken place, all have reported some improvements in acne with a low-GI diet, but only three of these showed scientifically significant improvements.[5] Those who benefited experienced improvements such as fewer acne breakouts, less oil production and smaller sebaceous glands (pores). In another US study, over 2,000 participants were placed on a low-GI diet for weight loss, and although the study didn't specifically look at acne, 87 per cent of patients experienced less acne following the low-GI diet, and 91 per cent said they needed less acne treatment.[6] With this in mind, let's look at how sugar and acne are connected.

How sugar contributes to acne

When we consume refined sugar such as a can of cola, our blood sugar levels spike quickly, causing a rapid rise in the hormone insulin, which is released to help our body manage those sugar levels, as well as the release of a second hormone called insulin-like growth factor (IGF-1). If you're susceptible, IGF-1 activates sebaceous glands in the skin and increases the production of oil (sebum), leading to congestion (hyperkeratinisation) and ultimately making skin more prone to breakouts.

As we have already learned in our discussion about AGEs (on page 61), sugar can also stiffen collagen fibres in the skin, and collagen is extremely important for skin healing and minimising scarring, so sticking to a lower GI diet may also help our skin recover from breakouts.

Polycystic ovarian syndrome (PCOS) and sugar

PCOS is a common hormonal imbalance that affects over 10 per cent of women. Acne can be the only outward sign of PCOS (another excellent example of the skin alerting us to other health conditions), but additional symptoms include irregular or absent periods, hair loss from the scalp, and increased unwanted hair growth on the face or body. The condition is characterised by high levels of insulin in the blood, which in turn causes elevated levels of androgen production and it is these hormones that are responsible for the outward symptoms of PCOS.

If these symptoms sound familiar in your case, do see your doctor to investigate further. It is important to make an early diagnosis, as there are specific treatment options for PCOS, and it may also be linked to other long-term health conditions; for example, the risk of developing type-2 diabetes and raised cholesterol. Finding out early means that you can make diet and lifestyle changes to reduce the chance of developing these conditions.

The SkinFood approach is an excellent way of eating if you have PCOS, as it contains dietary components that are key to managing symptoms, such as lower-GI carbohydrates to maintain insulin levels, omega-3-rich fish, healthy fats and plenty of fruit and veg.

Should I ditch the dairy?

For many of us, milk, cheese, butter and yoghurt are regularly found at mealtimes. Several studies, including one of the most reliable forms of research study known as a meta-analysis (essentially the combined results of many research studies), have found an association between drinking milk and the likelihood of developing acne. Researchers have concluded that people who drink two or more glasses of milk per day are more likely to suffer from breakouts,[7] with further studies suggesting that low-fat milk is more of a problem than full-fat milk. As yet, we don't have good enough evidence that other dairy foods such as yoghurt and cheese pose a problem.

How does dairy trigger acne?

There are many nutrients in dairy foods, and they are an excellent source of calcium – particularly for growing children and for reducing the risk of osteoporosis (a condition that weakens the bones) in women. Scientists believe that it is the hormone IGF-1, found naturally in dairy milk that is most likely the reason why it may trigger acne breakouts. Interestingly, the levels of IGF-1, a hormone that can contribute to increased sebum production and breakouts, are highest in skimmed milk and lower in cheese and yoghurt due to the way that these foods are processed. (Note that there is a common misconception that hormones added to milk cause acne. In the UK and the EU, dairy cows cannot be given hormones but, even so, milk from animals naturally contains several hormones in small amounts.)

Do you need to go dairy-free?

Nowadays, it seems that many people are experimenting with a dairy-free diet. But do you really need to? Dairy does have some nutritional benefits in that it contains vitamins and minerals such as calcium, B vitamins and iodine, plus it may well be something that you enjoy. Current research suggests that dairy milk, particularly skimmed milk, may contribute to acne for some people, particularly if they are drinking more than two glasses per day, but I don't think that this is enough for it to be necessary to completely exclude all dairy products such as cheese or yoghurt.

If you want to explore whether milk affects your skin further, I would try swapping dairy milk for a non-dairy alternative for 4 weeks to see if it makes a difference. It may also be helpful to take weekly photographs that can serve as a visual map of your skin's reaction to milk and, during this period, ensure that your skincare routine stays consistent, as introducing new products can aggravate your skin and will affect your research into the effects of the milk.

If you do notice an improvement, it's worth considering whether you want to continue avoiding dairy milk in the longer term. If that's the case, be careful to make up your daily calcium requirements using the information below.

Non-dairy alternatives In recent years there has been an explosion in the non-dairy market. There are now so many alternatives available that the choice can be overwhelming. Plant-based milks can differ quite considerably in their nutritional constituents, calcium and protein contents, as well as their GI, so I've compiled the table below to help you choose the right one for you.

I recommend looking for unsweetened options fortified with calcium, B12, B2, vitamin D and iodine where possible. My favourite in a coffee is oat milk, particularly as I like the way it froths in a cappuccino. It has a slightly higher GI than other alternatives, but I have it only once a day at most, and when I do it's in small quantities. If I'm making porridge or smoothies, my preference is to use fortified almond milk, as this has a lower GI and keeps my blood sugar steady. There are also environmental considerations when choosing plant milks so it's worth doing your homework on the impact of each before deciding which best meets your needs. To help make that decision a little easier, I've also included a nutritional breakdown of key alternatives in the table below:

Milk type	Calories Kcal/100ml	Protein/100ml	Calcium/100ml	B12/100ml	Glycaemic index
Full-fat cow's milk	66	3.5g	124µg	0.9mcg	35–40
Semi-skimmed cow's milk	50	3.6g	124µg	0.9mcg	35–40
Skimmed cow's milk	36	3.6g	130µg	0.9mcg	35–40
Alpro Soya Original	57	3.0g	120µg	0.38mcg	61.5
Alpro Soya Organic	32	3.3g	12.3µg	*	49.6
Oatly oat drink	46	1g	120µg	0.38µg	59.6

Rude Health organic brown rice drink	60	0.1g	*	*	99.96
Provamel organic almond drink	29	1.0g	*	*	64.2
Alpro Almond original	22	0.4g	120µg	0.38mcg	49.1
Alpro Coconut original	20	0.1g	120µg	0.38mcg	96.82
Alpro Hazelnut original	29	0.4g	120µg	0.38mcg	55.8

The differences between cow's milk and various milk alternatives.

* Denotes products that are not fortified with either calcium or B12 (Source: Jeske et al., 2016, Alpro.com, Rudehealth.com, Provamel.com, Tesco.com)

Other non-dairy calcium sources Adults in the UK require 700µg of calcium per day, while girls aged eleven to eighteen require 800µg per day and boys 1,000µg per day. Calcium is particularly important for bone development and preventing osteoporosis. As we have just learned, several plant-based milks are fortified with calcium, but there are other dairy-free sources that you can consider working into your diet to ensure that you maintain the recommended daily intake levels.

Product	Serving size	Calcium (µg)
Calcium-fortified soya, coconut or oat yoghurt	100g	120–211
Calcium-fortified coconut cheese	30g	45–221

Calcium-fortified cereals	30g	136–174
Sardines with bones in tomato sauce	60g (1/2 tin)	273–407
Fortified wholemeal bread	2 slices (100g)	106
Kale	100g boiled	150

The calcium quantities of certain foods.

Dietary supplements and acne

There are certain vitamins and supplements that can actually make acne worse. Over the last few years it's something I have seen more often due to the growing popularity of supplements. Here are some of the most common acne-aggravators:

- Whey protein supplements: whey is derived from dairy milk and contains high levels of IGF-1 that can worsen or trigger breakouts. Swap your whey for a plant-based alternative such as pea protein or brown rice protein.
- Vitamin B12: in the UK adults need only 1.5ug per day.
- Biotin supplements (B7): be careful with high doses of biotin (2,500µg and upwards) found in hair, skin and nail supplements.

On the flip side, there are also some supplements that may help acne:

- Vitamin D: make sure to take your daily requirement of vitamin D. Studies show that low levels can be linked to more significant acne. (I discussed vitamin D in detail on page 68.)
- Probiotics (see page 91).

- Inositol: a supplement that helps to regulate insulin. There is now good evidence that it can help PCOS and alleviate symptoms such as irregular periods as well as PCOS-related acne. A dose of 2g twice a day appears to be beneficial; look for a 40:1 ratio of the two types of inositol: myo-inositol to D-chiro-inositol. Keep in mind that it can take a few months to see the benefits. This should *not* be taken if you are pregnant. And, as always, do speak with your doctor first if you have any underlying medical conditions or you are taking medication regularly.

My top five foods for acne-prone skin

It's difficult to pick only five of the best foods for anyone with acne-prone skin, but I would say that the following are ones I recommend to all of my patients:

Flaxseeds	Rich in lignans that help to lower blood sugar and improve insulin resistance, and a good source of anti-inflammatory omega-3
Brown rice	Contains inositol, which helps to regulate blood sugar in PCOS
Walnuts	Contain ellagitannins, which are potent antioxidants that reduce inflammation
Probiotic foods	Such as kefir, kimchi and sauerkraut, which support gut bacteria particularly when taking acne treatments such as antibiotics
Green tea	Studies have shown it can reduce IGF-1 levels

Best foods for acne-prone skin.

Nutrition for radiant skin at any age

Decades of scientific research has pointed to several factors that determine how and when we develop fine lines, wrinkles, loss of plumpness, and discolouration, which can lead to an overall loss of vibrancy in the skin. Although premature ageing is not strictly a skin condition, it is something that I am asked about time and time again. Ageing is inevitable, but how we age is in our hands.

Intrinsic or biological ageing is down to our individual genes and the passage of time. Over the years, skin becomes thinner and increases in laxity, and the skin cells become sluggish and renew at a slower pace. Extrinsic ageing describes the many external factors our skin is exposed to that accelerate the ageing process and can leave it looking dull and lacklustre, but we have the power to address these external stressors through our diet and lifestyle, and in a moment we'll look at the most effective ways to do so.

Why diet matters

Sugar gets a bad rap, but not all sugar is bad. It is the processed and refined sugar found in sweet treats such as biscuits, cakes or fizzy drinks that we need to be mindful of, as when consumed in excess they can have a negative impact on our skin. We know that nutrients from the foods we eat reach the skin through the bloodstream, but when we consume excessive sugar, it can reach the dermis and form molecules called 'advanced glycation end products', appropriately known as AGEs, as previously discussed. AGEs damage collagen and elastin fibres, causing them to become stiff, therefore triggering inflammation and resulting in premature skin ageing that slows wound healing and repair. This discovery was first made in people who have diabetes, a condition caused by chronically high blood sugar levels. Studies have shown that those living with higher blood sugar can have thickened skin and appear visibly older than those with normal blood sugar levels.[8]

The ageing effect of sugar has come to be known as 'sugar sag'. As you know by now, I certainly don't believe in completely cutting out sugar, but there are ways in which we can indulge our sweet tooth that will have less of an impact on our blood sugar level, as we looked into in Chapter 4, and I've also included several of my favourite dessert recipes for you to try in Chapter 10. I can't stress enough that a balanced diet is integral to the SkinFood approach, and this includes moderating our sugar intake. Make sure to incorporate fibre-rich whole grains, protein, healthy fats and fresh fruit and vegetables in your diet, as they work in synergy to stabilise blood sugar and prevent sugar spikes.

Nutrition for radiant skin: berries before botox

In Skin School (Chapter 1) we learned how our skin loses radiance over time, due to a loss of collagen, the slower renewal rate of our cells, as well as DNA damage following years of exposure to sunlight and pollution. Good nutrition can profoundly impact how our skin looks and feels and the many aspects of how skin ages by counteracting several of the forces underlying internal and external ageing.

Ageing process	Nutrition target
Reactive oxygen species (ROS) or free radicals generated by UV light and pollution cause damage to collagen and accelerated ageing	A diet rich in vibrant-coloured fruit and vegetables, olive oil and green tea supplies the skin with antioxidants. Antioxidants work to counteract ROS and collagen damage.
Advance glycation end products (AGEs) stiffen collagen causing skin to lose elasticity and tone	AGEs occur as a result of sugar molecules such as glucose and fructose from the food we eat, so limiting refined sugars and keeping blood sugar levels stable can help to counteract this. AGEs are also found in high levels in fried foods, so it is best to limit these where possible
Chronic low-grade inflammation is a characteristic of ageing known as 'inflammageing'	Omega-3, vitamins A, C, D and E and green tea provide anti-inflammatory benefits. Intermittent fasting has also been shown to have anti-inflammatory effects on the body (in human studies) and increased longevity (in mice studies)
Cells divide less frequently due to telomere shortening (see page 36)	Optimising the gut microbiome has been shown to help preserve telomere length

Good nutrition and the ageing process.

The SkinFood approach outlined in Chapter 4 has been precisely developed to incorporate all the elements required for optimal ageing and is based on research studies; for example:

- Research has shown that a high intake of vegetables, oily fish, olive oil, beans and pulses protect against skin ageing, whereas a diet rich in dairy and butter appeared to show the opposite.[9]
- A study of over 4,000 American women between the ages of 40 and 74 found that those who ate a diet rich in the antioxidant vitamin C and omega fatty acids were found to have skin that appeared to age better compared to those who consumed more fats and carbohydrates.[10]
- A 15-year study of 700 Australian adults found that those who ate a diet rich in antioxidants aged significantly better than those who did not.[11]
- A study of 700 Japanese women found that those who ate more green and yellow vegetables had fewer wrinkles than those who didn't.[12]

Focus on filling your plate with whole grains, colourful fruit and vegetables, lean protein and healthy fats for skin health (as shown on the plate on page 112). As we learned in Chapter 4, these foods truly are nutrient powerhouses. Keeping a steady weight and avoiding yo-yo dieting is also key to optimising our skin health, as fluctuations in weight can stretch the skin, making it less elastic and more likely to sag.

Nutrition for the menopause

During the perimenopause and menopause, skin can start to become dry and lose radiance. This is when signs of premature skin ageing can become more prominent. As oestrogen levels slowly decline, symptoms such as hot flushes and irregular periods start to occur, as well as a myriad of other symptoms. These hormonal changes can also impact the skin, contributing to acne breakouts and a loss of collagen. This is because oestrogen helps the skin to regulate oil production and retain collagen in the skin. The SkinFood approach will support skin health during this time of life but there are additional ways that we can use nutrition to our advantage. Plants contain a naturally occurring form of oestrogen called phytoestrogen. Eating foods rich in phytoestrogen might help to alleviate some of the symptoms of the menopause, but it is more effective to try to include plant oestrogens several times throughout the day rather than in one go. Here are some of the best plant sources of phytoestrogen:

- Flaxseeds – lignans in these foods function as phytoestrogen.
- Soya beans, edamame and tofu – these foods can also help to improve the symptoms of hot flushes.
- Prioritise bone health by regularly incorporating calcium-rich foods (page 150).
- Consider trying collagen supplements (more on this below); you'd need to try these for about 12 weeks to see any benefits.

If you're struggling with perimenopausal breakouts, you're certainly not alone. I will offer additional ways to support your skin when we explore Step 3 and Step 4 of the 4-Step Skin Solution.

*

As a general rule, I try to incorporate the foods in the table below into my meals on a regular basis, but if you have an important occasion coming up, ensure that you're consuming these foods daily for a few weeks before your big event to maximise skin benefits.

Here are my top beauty foods for healthy ageing:

Blackberries	Contain the highest levels of antioxidants of all berries
Walnuts	Contain omega-3 and ellagic acid, a potent antioxidant
Green tea	Rich in catechins, which improve antioxidant activity
Green leafy vegetables	Kale, spinach and other greens contain high levels of lutein and zeaxanthin, which protect against UV damage and can help to even skin tone and enhance overall brightness when taken as supplements
Salmon	Omega-3s found in oily fish have anti-inflammatory benefits. Salmon also contains astaxanthin, responsible for its pink colour, which improves skin hydration and elasticity
Tomatoes	Contain lycopene, which mop up damaging free radicals within the skin

The top beauty foods.

Supplements for healthy skin ageing

By now you'll be familiar with my ethos that real food should be our primary source of nutrients, but there can be phases in our life when this is a challenge and we turn to supplements; for example, it might be that you've had a hectic week at work and your food choices haven't been what you'd like them to be.

Taking a good-quality multivitamin is perfectly reasonable, as long as you remember that nutrition isn't about what we eat over a few days or even weeks – it is about our overall pattern of eating.

The following is a list of the supplements that I am most frequently asked about in relation to radiance and premature skin ageing.

Collagen supplements

As we know, collagen is the most abundant protein in the skin, but as levels of it drop over time our skin loses its elasticity. There are numerous collagen supplements marketed to target exactly this problem, but are they the miracle anti-ageing supplements they are claimed to be? Let's look at the science before I answer this question.

As I outlined earlier, collagen is a huge protein molecule, supported by strong bonds that give our skin its resilience. Collagen supplements do not contain collagen molecules; instead, they contain fragments of collagen peptides, made up of short chains of amino acids. When we eat proteins, they are digested and broken down into individual amino acids, which are absorbed into the bloodstream to be used where they are needed.

You would think, therefore, that collagen peptides would just be broken down into their constituent amino acids following digestion, but studies have shown that collagen peptides are found in the blood of people who have been given collagen supplements. We aren't quite sure how this works, although it is intriguing nonetheless. Research is also yet to ascertain whether these collagen peptides in the blood eventually make it to the skin, or whether they are simply distributed throughout the body. What we do know is that certain collagen peptides have been used as a skincare ingredient for decades, and when tested in the laboratory studies show that these peptides or collagen fragments can encourage fibroblasts in the skin to make more collagen.

Although we still cannot be sure how collagen supplements work, the evidence from published clinical trials seems to support the theory that they could be beneficial. A review of nineteen studies that looked at the effects of collagen supplements was published in 2021 and found that almost all studies showed improved skin elasticity, hydration and reduced facial wrinkles – and, importantly, no adverse effects were reported.[13] It should be noted, though, that the studies used different collagen formulations (beef, fish, chicken) for varying doses and durations, which makes comparisons between studies less accurate. The vast majority of the studies published were funded by collagen supplement manufacturers, so the results ought to be taken with a pinch of salt. The question also remains about whether we are simply providing our body with an additional amino acid/protein source by consuming collagen supplements that we could get by eating more protein instead.

What then is my advice? If collagen supplements are something you are intrigued by, it is worth giving them a go for 3 months and stopping if you don't see an improvement, as there is very little to lose. I have tried collagen supplements myself over the years and I have personally found them to improve my skin's hydration. If you are going to try a collagen supplement, look for ones containing type-1 collagen (found in the skin) with dipeptides (such as proline-hydroxyproline or hydroxyproline-glycine) as these appear to show faster clinical results in studies. From the limited studies available it is difficult to determine whether fish- or meat-derived collagen are superior, and as such this is a matter of personal preference. Vegan collagen peptides are also available, but there is less research on their effectiveness. Liquid formulations and collagen drinks are more expensive, but as far as the current research goes, they don't offer a superior advantage. You should know that in order to make collagen, your body requires both iron and vitamin C, so make sure you include adequate amounts of both of these in your diet or supplement appropriately.

Polypodium leucotomos extract

I first discovered this supplement, extracted from a Central American fern plant, when tackling my own sun sensitivity. Known as Fernblock™, this particular antioxidant and anti-inflammatory supplement increases the skin's ability to withstand the harmful effects of UV light. It quenches free radicals and prevents DNA damage and can help those of us with sun-sensitive skin (but note that it does not replace sunscreen). Clinical trials show that it can also protect against UV-induced skin ageing. This is a more costly supplement, so I usually recommend it only if you have sun-sensitive skin, either due to a fair skin tone or a medical condition, but in my experience it really does work.

Vitamin C

You might remember that we looked at vitamin C supplementation in Chapter 2, so if you're interested in this area, turn back to pages 75–8.

Alcohol and skin ageing

Alcohol is ageing for our skin, and can flare skin conditions such as rosacea, eczema and psoriasis. That doesn't mean that you can't enjoy it, but be mindful of how much you're consuming and how often. In the clinic, I recommend cutting back on alcohol as much as possible if you are trying to get your skin in shape for a big event, and I often advise models, actresses or brides to cut back completely in the 2 weeks before a photoshoot or wedding. It might sound boring, but it really does work.

When you do drink, choose red wine if you can (as long as it doesn't flare up any co-existing skin concerns such as rosacea). You might be wondering what's so special about red wine, and this is down to how it's made. Red wine (unlike white) is produced using the skin of the grapes, and these contain a powerful antioxidant called resveratrol. It is thought that this is why occasional glasses of red wine are also good for the heart.

Research studies have reinforced my own observations that alcohol can make us age prematurely. One study noted that drinking more alcohol, defined as greater than eight alcoholic drinks per week, was associated with increased upper facial lines, under-eye puffiness, loss of facial volume and visible blood vessels.[14] Alcohol can impair the skin's antioxidant defence system, hastening the ageing process and leaving skin looking dull. Try cutting back for a couple of weeks to see if you notice any difference in your skin.

Nutrition for rosacea

I like to divide the role of nutrition in rosacea into two categories: (1) finding your personal triggers; and (2) gut health and the role of the gut microbiome.

If you have rosacea, the best place to start is by finding your personal triggers. Once you identify them, they don't have to rule your life; instead work with them and have flexibility without being restrictive. If you love red wine but it sets your skin off, choose when you want to enjoy that glass or two. If it's coffee you're craving, allow it to cool a little or go for an iced option instead. From my experience in the clinic, rosacea responds beautifully to the 4-Step Skin Solution, so it's all about choosing the right skincare and medical treatments, diligently protecting against the sun and addressing food and lifestyle triggers to achieve long-term control and confidence.

Trigger warning

If you have rosacea, you are probably already familiar with certain triggers that cause your skin to flare up. Saying that, I have met patients who have lived with rosacea for years and were still surprised to find out that their favourite tipple was actually making their skin condition markedly worse. For some people the face will feel warm, tingly and flushed within minutes of drinking a glass of wine, whereas for others it's a spicy curry that will set their skin off. Although there is a great deal of variability, a survey of over 1,000 people with rosacea reported that the following are the most common triggers people experience:

- Sun exposure (81 per cent)
- Emotional stress (79 per cent)
- Heavy exercise (56 per cent)
- Alcohol (52 per cent)
- Spicy food (45 per cent)
- Hot drinks (36 per cent)

I find it more helpful to group rosacea triggers into the broad categories that I've outlined in the table below. As you read through this list, I want you to keep in mind that only *some* of these triggers will apply to you, certainly not all.

Category	Examples
Emotional	Stress Anxiety Embarrassment
Environment	UV light Wind Cold weather
Activities	Strenuous exercise Saunas and steam rooms Hot yoga Smoking
Skincare product ingredients	Physical exfoliants such as grainy scrubs Some hydroxy acids (for example, AHA and BHAs) Alcohol and acetone Menthol, camphor and fragrances Benzalkonium chloride and propylene glycol Sodium lauryl sulphate
Foods (see also page 168)	Spicy food Cinnamaldehyde-containing foods (for example, cinnamon, tomatoes, citrus and chocolate) Fermented/aged foods
Drinks (see also page 167)	Hot beverages Alcohol (wine, beer)
Hormones	Pregnancy, menopause

Common rosacea triggers.

It's important to remember that these triggers don't actually cause rosacea, but they can add fuel to the fire and aggravate flare-ups. By keeping track of potential triggers through a rosacea trigger diary (see Resources for a link to an online template), you can begin to pinpoint what factors might set off your skin. I recommend keeping the diary for around 2 weeks to see if you spot any patterns. It should be fairly easy to narrow down whether a specific food or ingredient is a trigger for you, as rosacea symptoms typically flare quite quickly, almost always within 30 minutes. If you are still struggling to pinpoint which foods are causing flare-ups, I recommend speaking to your doctor or a dietitian, who can support you.

An important point to stress is that you do not need to cut out all of these triggers to keep rosacea under control. The purpose of this table and the rosacea diary is to identify the triggers that are unique to you. No two people with rosacea have the same triggers, but being aware of your own will put you in the driver's seat and help you to keep your skin under control. A study by the National Rosacea Society found that almost three-quarters of people who made tweaks to their diet successfully reduced flare-ups.

Like many skin conditions, rosacea is a complex culmination of genetics, our environment and lifestyle, as we'll see now in Patrick's case.

CASE STUDY: BEING IN CONTROL OF YOUR SKIN

Patrick was a high-flying investment banker, who had been prone to rosacea for many years. He came to see me after his skin took a turn for the worse. His redness had become more troublesome and he had started to develop spots and raised red areas on his cheeks too. It affected his confidence at work, particularly when he was dealing with clients. I asked him about any recent changes to his lifestyle, and he acknowledged that he was under more stress, entertaining clients regularly, drinking more alcohol than he used to, and that he'd started drinking endless cups of hot coffee to help battle the long hours.

To address Patrick's rosacea, I asked him to complete a rosacea trigger diary, which we then reviewed together before designing a tailored plan based on the 4-Step Skin Solution that would help to keep his flare-ups at bay.

- **Step 1** We addressed Patrick's food choices when eating out with clients, and I encouraged him to avoid those spices that would cause him to flush, such as chilli and cayenne pepper. In addition, I introduced him to the core elements of the SkinFood approach and encouraged him to reduce his overall alcohol consumption as well as to try alternatives to red wine that are less likely to cause flare-ups, such as vodka. I also suggested that he allow his coffee to cool to room temperature before drinking it.
- **Step 2** We began by talking about stress management. I am a huge fan of meditation, so we discussed apps that he could use to incorporate this habit into Patrick's daily life.
- **Step 3** I then introduced him to a simple skincare routine, with ingredients targeted at redness, and I combined this with an invisible mineral-based, high-factor sunscreen.
- **Step 4** In Patrick's case, medical treatment wasn't required because he responded so well to Steps 1 to 3.

He felt confident in managing his symptoms in the longer term, and this allowed him to feel in control of his skin, rather than feeling that his skin was controlling him.

How to manage triggers

There are several ways to manage rosacea triggers, but the first thing to do is to consider which foods and drinks might be causing your skin to flare up so that you can make effective changes to your diet.

Alcohol

Alcohol is often linked to rosacea flare-ups. A study of over 80,000 women found that those who drank alcohol were at greater risk of developing rosacea.[15] This is because alcoholic beverages contain varying levels of a compound called histamine, which is produced during the fermentation process. Our body produces histamine naturally in small amounts, but for some people with rosacea, histamine causes blood vessels in the skin to widen and increases the appearance of redness and flushing.

Red wine is the most notorious culprit for aggravating redness, as it contains the highest levels of histamine. Prosecco, cava and dry white wines such as Sauvignon Blanc are marginally better choices. This is because histamine is found at higher levels in grape skin, and red wine is made with the whole grape. For white wine, the skin is separated from the juice before the fermentation process. Beer also contains higher levels of histamines due to the way in which it is fermented. Clear liquors such as tequila, gin and vodka have the lowest levels of histamine, so these make better alternatives – but as always remember to consume them in moderation.

There is a misconception that rosacea is aggravated by drinking *too much* alcohol – for some of my patients just a few sips can be enough to trigger flushing.

Fermented and aged foods

Histamine is a by-product of food fermentation by bacteria and yeasts. High-histamine foods include aged cheeses such as Parmesan, Cheddar and blue cheese, plus fermented foods such as sauerkraut, kimchi and kefir. Processed meats like ham and salami also contain high levels of histamines.

You can again use the trigger diary to monitor whether any of these foods are an issue for you. If they do cause your skin to flare up, think about reducing the amounts you eat. If you know you're going to be eating a meal containing problematic high-histamine foods once in a while, you could consider taking an over-the-counter antihistamine tablet about 2 hours before you eat. Please remember that some antihistamines can make you sleepy, so it is best not to combine them with alcoholic drinks or driving.

Spices

Piquant spices such as chilli and cayenne pepper can aggravate redness, as they contain a compound called capsaicin, which gives them their spicy flavour. Capsaicin can stimulate nerve endings to produce inflammation in the skin that subsequently leads to flushing and redness. If you love spicy food, try dialling down the heat to prevent flares.

Another trigger is cinnamaldehyde, a compound that gives cinnamon its distinctive flavour, which can cause a warming sensation and trigger rosacea symptoms. In addition to cinnamon, you can find cinnamaldehyde in tomatoes, citrus fruits (such as lemons and limes) and chocolate. You'll be pleased to hear that, in my experience, these foods don't tend to pose as much of a problem, so it might be that smaller amounts are tolerable for you.

Hot drinks

Although coffee and tea are often blamed for rosacea flare-ups, recent studies have shown that it is not caffeine that's the problem but the temperature at which you drink it. Researchers found that allowing coffee to cool down meant that it was much less likely to flare redness than when drinking it while it is piping hot. Make sure therefore to let your cup cool down to room temperature before drinking to fend off flares.

What should I eat if I have rosacea?

The anti-inflammatory SkinFood approach is an ideal place to start when eating to support rosacea. Where possible, focus on supporting good gut health, because as we learned in Chapter 3 there is a fascinating link between gut health and rosacea. The following foods have particular benefits:

Oily fish, walnuts, flaxseeds	Rich in omega-3 to support the skin barrier
Green tea (cool)	High in antioxidants
Dark coloured berries	Rich in anthocyanin antioxidants
Probiotic foods	Increase diversity of good bacteria in the GM
Prebiotic foods	Feed good bacteria

Nutrition for psoriasis

If you have ever wondered if diet plays a role in psoriasis, you are certainly not alone. In fact, this is the number-one question for people living with psoriasis – and it's actually the question that led me to studying nutrition in the first place. My initial curiosity, piqued by talking to patients, evolved into a passion, and, as mentioned previously, I'm now part of a King's College research team that is working to uncover the links between diet and psoriasis in a ground-breaking project known as the APPLE Study (Asking People with Psoriasis about Lifestyle and Eating),[16] which is funded by the Psoriasis Association in the UK. Our research team includes internationally renowned dermatologist, Professor Christopher Griffiths and nutrition scientists – a first for a study in the UK.

If you have psoriasis, nutrition matters for several reasons. Firstly, psoriasis isn't just a skin condition, it is closely linked to several other medical conditions. Studies have shown that people with psoriasis have a higher risk of developing other long-term health conditions such as: heart disease, type-2 diabetes, high blood pressure and high cholesterol. But please don't be alarmed, as the good news is that all these conditions respond very well to changes in diet and lifestyle, so taking care of your health is essential. Not only can it prevent the occurrence of these linked conditions, but it can also improve psoriasis itself.

In recent years we have learned that psoriasis might also be linked to carrying extra body weight. I know that weight is an emotionally charged issue, so I've thought long and hard about including it in this section, but it wouldn't be fair not to discuss it. I want to give you all the information and evidence that's available so that you can make your own empowered decisions.

Research indicates that people who experience excess body weight are more likely to have psoriasis and to have a more severe form of the condition. We think it is because the cells that store fat in the body, known as adipose cells, can drive further inflammation. Studies also suggest that carrying extra weight reduces the effectiveness of several treatments used for psoriasis and increases the risk of developing linked conditions such as type-2 diabetes.

Many studies have also looked at the effect of weight loss on the severity of psoriasis in people who are overweight or who live with obesity. The overall finding shows that with as little as a 5 per cent reduction in body weight psoriasis improves.[17] Weight loss also appears to reduce the amount of medical treatment required to keep psoriasis under control. Up to one-third of people with psoriasis also have a type of arthritis known as psoriatic arthritis, and weight loss seems to play an important role in managing this too, as it helps take pressure off swollen or tender joints. It is important to stress that these research studies show that weight loss only benefits those psoriasis patients whose weight is elevated. If your weight lies within a healthy range, additional weight loss is not recommended, but following the balanced SkinFood approach will still be beneficial.

Living with obesity is influenced by many factors, including the environment and social factors, as well as our individual biology. If you are looking to lose weight, I urge you to seek the help of a doctor or dietitian to support you in your journey, as it will help the chance of long-term success hugely. In the clinic, I work with experienced dietitians who offer support for people who wish to make such changes. It's not simply a matter of eating less and moving more, it's about creating the right environment and offering psychological support so that changes can happen more easily.

CASE STUDY: A HEALTHIER DIET HELPS PSORIASIS

Sophie was in her thirties when she first came to see me. She had developed psoriasis in her early twenties, with red, scaly patches on her arms, legs and scalp. Not only was it painful and itchy, but she also felt embarrassed by her skin. Too ashamed to go swimming or to the beach, Sophie's confidence had hit rock bottom. Although she used to love going out with her friends, as her psoriasis had worsened, she had become more withdrawn. This had led Sophie to try lots of different creams and ointments, but none of these offered the sustained relief that she was looking for.

We talked about Sophie's lifestyle, including her diet, exercise habits and alcohol intake. It turned out that she had stopped exercising and her diet had gradually changed over the years, with her meals often consisting of takeaways in the evenings with a few glasses of wine. Her weight had slowly crept up and she felt uncomfortable in her clothes. Sophie had started to wonder whether her weight was impacting her psoriasis, as she had noticed that it had worsened alongside her weight increase.

After our initial conversation, I carried out tests to check Sophie's liver, blood pressure, cholesterol and to see whether type-2 diabetes could be a factor. When her results returned, I was concerned to see that her levels of harmful cholesterol, known as LDL (low-density lipoprotein), were high. Elevated levels of LDL can increase the risk of heart attacks and strokes over time, so we implemented the 4-Step Skin Solution and addressed changes that would help Sophie, starting with the SkinFood approach:

- **Step 1** We focused on incorporating nutritious colourful fruits and vegetables into her day: porridge with berries and seeds for breakfast; olive oil on salads; and healthier takeaway options, as well as easy batch-cooking meals for the weekend.
- **Step 2** Sophie also started walking more as both a mindfulness practice and to improve her fitness and cutting back on her alcohol intake.

These simple tweaks to her lifestyle allowed her to feel better in herself and more positive and confident. As well as reducing her cholesterol levels, her skin improved too, and the remaining patches of psoriasis could be treated with:

- **Step 3** A calming skincare routine to reduce itching and irritation.
- **Step 4** A Vitamin D prescription cream to improve scaling and inflammation.

By changing her daily habits, Sophie not only took care of her skin but also lowered her overall risk of developing other chronic health conditions. Sophie's story is just one of so many I could share from the psoriasis clinic. Being mindful of nutrition should be an absolute priority if you have psoriasis, both for your skin and your long-term health.

Common questions from the clinic

In this section I'll answer some of the most common questions I get asked in the clinic to help guide you through the latest science relating to psoriasis.

Q: 'Do I need to go on a juice cleanse, a detox, or an elimination diet?'
A: No! As I've mentioned already, I firmly believe that you do not need to follow an extreme diet to help your skin. Such diets are not sustainable in the long term and can make you miserable. As with other skin conditions we've covered, maintaining a healthy diet and reducing inflammatory, heavily processed foods, rather than eliminating food groups, is the best way forward. From my experience, there is no hard and fast rule when it comes to trigger foods, and instead it can vary from person to person. However, a survey conducted in the US of over 1,000 people with psoriasis found that the following foods were reported to cause flares: sugar, alcohol, tomato, gluten and dairy.[18] In addition, I always advise keeping alcohol intake to a minimum and being mindful of refined sugar too. If you think dairy could be influencing your psoriasis, then you may consider removing it from your diet for a period of 4 weeks to see if you notice any improvement. On page 148 we explore how to do this safely and optimise dairy-free calcium sources. If you don't see an improvement after the 4-week period, do remember to re-introduce dairy at the end.

Q: 'Should I go gluten-free?'
A: Many patients (and colleagues!) have asked this question, and here is my science-backed answer. Research has shown that if you have coeliac disease or a positive coeliac blood test (performed by

your doctor rather than self-administered tests purchased online), going gluten-free can help to improve psoriasis.[19] Coeliac disease is an immune condition that affects 1 in 100 people in the UK in which the body attacks the gluten protein found in wheat, resulting in inflammation in the gut that causes bloating, pain and diarrhoea. Coeliac disease is about three times more common if you already have psoriasis, so if you have ever suffered from any of these symptoms, make sure to see your doctor to test for coeliac disease. It's important that you don't cut gluten out of your diet before the test is done, as this can invalidate the results.

Cutting out gluten doesn't seem to help if you don't fall into the above categories. As we have seen, some gluten-free foods can be more expensive and more heavily processed than their gluten-containing counterparts, so do not feel that you have to cut out gluten, especially as it isn't automatically a healthier option.

Q: 'Should I go vegan?'
A: I fully support people who follow a vegan diet, but if your sole purpose in doing so is to help clear your psoriasis, it wouldn't be my first-choice recommendation, as there isn't evidence that suggests it has an effect. Plant-based diets, however, tend to have fewer processed foods and saturated fats and can help with weight management so they can still be beneficial to your health. Eating a wide variety of fruit, vegetables and whole grains also helps our good gut bacteria to thrive. If you are going to follow a vegan diet, see my tips on page 82 to make sure you get all the nutrients you need.

Q: 'Should I avoid nightshades?'
A: Nightshades are a group of plants containing compounds called alkaloids, which can be a problem in people with inflammatory

bowel disease. These foods include: aubergines, peppers, potatoes and tomatoes.

Some people with psoriasis report that eating these foods causes their skin to flare, but the link between these foods and psoriasis hasn't been studied yet. From my perspective, I have not found that removing nightshades from the diet to be particularly helpful to my psoriasis patients, but your experience may differ. There are many health benefits to these foods (for example, tomatoes contain the antioxidant lycopene, and peppers are rich in vitamin C) so I don't advocate excluding them unnecessarily; however, if you personally experience symptoms after consuming any of these foods, by all means omit them for a period of 4 weeks to see if you notice any improvement – but don't forget to reintroduce them at the end of the trial period if your psoriasis is unchanged.

How the SkinFood approach can help with psoriasis

Research has shown that people who follow a Mediterranean diet are likely to have milder psoriasis, and this style of eating is widely considered optimal for heart health, so it also helps to address long-term health conditions that might be linked to psoriasis. As the SkinFood approach is a skin-focused evolution of the Mediterranean approach to food it comes with all the same benefits with added skin love! Here are five of my top foods for psoriasis:

Olive oil	Linked to less severe psoriasis
Oily fish	Rich in anti-inflammatory omega-3 and associated with less severe psoriasis
Whole grains	Lower risk of high cholesterol and heart disease
Probiotic foods	Such as kimchi, kefir and kombucha to support the gut microbiome

Turmeric	A potent anti-inflammatory spice

The best foods to treat psoriasis.

Intermittent fasting

I'm not going to go into too much detail here, as I explained the many benefits of intermittent fasting and its connection to psoriasis in Chapter 4, but essentially it has anti-inflammatory health benefits, and it can also help with weight loss. If you have psoriasis, I would recommend trying it for 1 month to see if it works for you.

Alcohol

Alcohol can have an adverse effect on psoriasis, as it increases inflammation, and it can also prevent some medical treatments from working effectively. If you're regularly consuming alcohol in larger quantities, I would recommend speaking to your doctor, as it could be negatively affecting your skin. My recommendation is to be very mindful of how much alcohol you drink if you have psoriasis and to keep it to an absolute minimum. The UK Guidance allows a maximum of fourteen units spread over a week, amounting to six medium (175ml) glasses of wine, but I would try to stick well below this. Red wine has additional health benefits for the heart, so a couple of glasses a week should not be a problem.

Supplements

Vitamin D Psoriasis often improves with sunshine, and studies have shown that people with the condition have lower vitamin D levels than people who don't. Be sure to supplement during the winter months or year-round if you don't expose your skin to the sun much or have a deeper skin tone (see page 85 for dosing).

Omega-3 As omega-3 has many anti-inflammatory benefits, I recommend taking 500µg EPA/DHA per day if you don't eat oily fish at least twice a week or you are vegan.

Proanthocyanidin extract Currently, I am interested in a type of antioxidant called grapeseed proanthocyanidin extract. In early laboratory studies performed in mice, this has been shown to reduce the type of inflammation found in psoriasis.[20] It is a supplement that is generally considered safe, with very few side effects in humans (but should be avoided in pregnancy/breast-feeding). I look forward to the results of studies in people who have psoriasis before we draw firm conclusions.

Key skin-friendly takeaways

There are specific tweaks to the SkinFood approach that can help with acne, skin ageing, psoriasis and rosacea:

1. Dairy, particularly low-fat milk and high-glycaemic index foods, can trigger acne breakouts *for some.*

2. Radiant, youthful skin starts on your plate, remember: berries before botox.

3. Nutrition should be central to the management of psoriasis and linked conditions.

4. Identifying your personal triggers and optimising gut health will help to keep rosacea in check.

6

Eczema, Food Allergies and Intolerances

If you have eczema, there is no doubt that you've wondered whether food may be playing a role. In Chapter 1 we learned about what causes eczema, and how our genes and the skin barrier are a crucial factor driving eczema flare-ups.

It can be tricky to work out what causes eczema flare-ups, as eczema is by its very nature one of the most unpredictable skin conditions. One day your skin might be calm, and the next it's angry and itchy. It is because of such fluctuations that so many people look to food as a possible cause. There is so much confusion around food and eczema, so let's get to work on clearing it up.

What are food allergies?

Firstly, when we talk about food allergies, what do we actually mean? A food allergy is caused by our immune system reacting to a food that we have eaten; however, the confusion often arises because there are other types of reactions to food that can easily be mistaken for an allergy. The illustration below shows these different types of reaction, and we will explore how you can tell the difference between them.

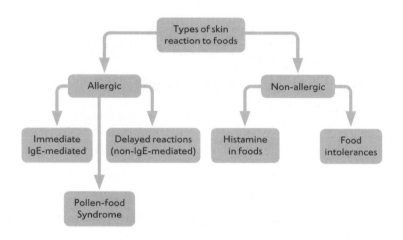

Different types of reactions to food seen in eczema can be divided into allergic and non-allergic reactions. Allergic reactions can be further divided into two subtypes.

It's perfectly possible to have food allergies without any underlying eczema. And there are many people with eczema who don't have food allergies.

The majority of studies looking at food allergies and eczema have focused on children, and there is less information available when looking at adults. Up to one in five children who have eczema may also have a food allergy. This does not necessarily mean that the food allergy is driving their eczema.

From my experience, although food allergies can be present in adults with eczema, they are much less common than in children. I frequently encounter adults, however, who try to cure their eczema by looking for a food allergy as the cause. It can be frustrating when allergy tests return as negative. This is because there are many other triggers for eczema flare-ups that are likely to be more relevant for adults, including:

- Stress – emotional stress is an important trigger for flare-ups and itching.
- Irritants in skincare products such as soaps, bubble bath and detergents.
- Environmental allergens particularly house dust mite (the commonest allergen for people with eczema), mould, pollen.
- Hormonal changes – eczema can flare up before the menstrual cycle and during/after pregnancy or around the menopause.
- Changes in weather, temperature and humidity.

You can treat eczema by sticking to an effective skincare routine, using prescription treatments if needed and avoiding triggers (Steps 3 and 4) and minimising other triggers such as stress (Step 2). As food allergies are rarely the sole driver of adult eczema, we would only look for them if your eczema did not improve with standard treatment.

How do I know if I have a food allergy?

Do food allergies cause eczema? Does everyone with eczema have a food allergy? What's a food intolerance? These are some of the many questions I'm asked in the clinic.

Firstly, food allergies occur when the body recognises something that should be harmless (food) as a potential threat. This results in an inappropriate immune reaction that can result in a range of possible symptoms:

- Anaphylaxis: a severe allergic reaction that causes swelling of the tongue and throat and impairs breathing – this is the most severe form of allergy and can be life threatening.
- Hives or urticaria: swollen lumps or welts on the skin.
- Itching of the skin.
- Stomach upset such as vomiting or diarrhoea.
- Flare-up of existing eczema.

Why are people with eczema more prone to food allergies? Although food allergies themselves do not usually cause eczema in adults, they can occasionally trigger flare-ups. The more severe the eczema, the higher the risk of developing food allergies. It is therefore very important to keep eczema under control.

If children unnecessarily avoid eating certain foods when they are young, it can actually increase their chance of developing an allergy to that food later in life. A landmark study known as LEAP (Learning Early about Peanut Allergy) showed that regularly eating peanuts early in life could prevent children from developing a peanut allergy;[1] however, if your child has a high risk of food allergies (for example there is a family history of reactions), then consult your doctor or dietitian on how to introduce high-allergy foods. To learn more, visit the Allergy UK website (see Resources).

Types of food allergy

Food allergies are often divided into two broad categories: immediate (IgE-mediated) and delayed (non-IgE mediated) reactions. In the table below you will find the crucial differences between these types of reaction.

Immediate reaction	Delayed reaction
Usually happens quickly, within minutes to hours of eating the trigger food	Symptoms can take up to 48 hours to appear
Can cause hives, tongue and lip swelling, worsening eczema, difficulty breathing, vomiting and diarrhoea	A less severe reaction that can flare pre-existing eczema
Can be life-threatening and may require an adrenaline EpiPen to be carried	Eczema flare-ups can be treated with creams or medications
Specific allergy tests can be used to help make the diagnosis	There are no specific tests for making the diagnosis. Instead, we use supervised elimination from the diet of particular foods and then gradual re-introduction to see if there is a relationship
Can occur whether eczema is under control or not – trigger food must be completely avoided at all times.	Trigger foods may be tolerated better when eczema is under control

The different allergic reactions.

If you think you may have a food allergy, it's essential that you speak with your doctor.

Immediate reactions

The most severe form of allergic reaction is an anaphylactic reaction. If you have an allergy to peanuts, for example, even eating a trace can lead to rapid swelling of the lips, tongue and throat leading to difficulty breathing. Without a doubt this is the most dangerous and life-threatening type of food allergy.

Immediate allergic reactions aren't always this dramatic. Immediate allergies can also appear as hives or urticaria (swollen, often burning areas of skin that resemble nettle rash) and itching. Sometimes they can cause stomach upsets such as vomiting or diarrhoea too. In some cases, reactions can also appear as worsening of eczema, usually within hours.

The following foods are most commonly responsible for immediate allergic reactions:

Eggs
Milk and dairy products
Nuts and seeds
Shellfish and fish
Soy products
Wheat

If you suffer from this type of allergy (or you are the parent/carer of someone who does), it can be daunting trying to work out how to avoid trigger foods, particularly when it comes to eating out. I strongly advise that you seek help from a specialist allergy dietitian, who can share advice on how to go about navigating food choices (see Resources for tips on how to find a dietitian).

Delayed reactions

Delayed reactions are trickier to unpick. These types of reaction can cause flare-ups of pre-existing eczema. The reaction can occur several hours or even days (although usually within 48 hours) after the trigger food was eaten. The main challenge is that because there is a time delay it is harder to work out which food is responsible. It is likely that several different foods may have been eaten in the intervening time. Delayed reactions are also more variable in nature: sometimes they can cause severe eczema flare-ups, and at other times milder reactions. This inconsistency also makes it difficult to pinpoint a cause.

What makes things even harder is that, unlike immediate reactions, we don't have useful tests that help us to confirm the potential allergen. This is because we still don't fully understand exactly how the immune system causes this type of reaction to occur. This can be frustrating, and often some detective work is needed to find the problematic food or foods. In such situations, we turn to a systematic process to explore possible causes:

1 Observe and record all foods that are eaten over a specified time frame and eczema symptoms (usually over a 2-week period).
2 Identify if any food(s) are associated with flare-ups of eczema.
3 Omit those foods from the diet for a period of time (less than 4 weeks) to monitor for any improvement.
4 Gradually reintroduce the food(s) one at a time and check for signs of eczema flares.

This process is best undertaken with the support of a specialist dietitian. The most common trigger foods for delayed reactions are similar to those for immediate reactions:

Cow's milk
Eggs
Peanuts
Wheat

One interesting phenomenon that I have noticed with delayed reactions, particularly in adults, is that when eczema is better controlled, for example with creams or medical treatments, foods that previously caused delayed reactions seem to have less of an impact. This is why treating eczema should take a holistic approach, incorporating all four steps of the Skin Solution.

How to test for food allergies (and how not to)

In the clinic, if I suspect that someone has a food allergy, I don't hesitate to refer them on to a specialist allergy doctor for further investigation. This is because food allergies need to be diagnosed carefully to prevent the unnecessary restriction of food groups, which can actually increase the risk of developing allergies later in life. Allergy specialists are skilled detectives, asking detailed questions to find out which foods (if any) could be driving allergies and then arranging for investigations to explore this further. Such investigations include:

- Specific IgE blood test – this looks at whether the body is producing an immune reaction to certain foods.
- Skin-prick testing – a small amount of an allergen, for example peanut, is applied into the skin with a tiny needle to see if it causes a reaction.
- Oral food challenge – a small amount of the food is

given by mouth (in a safe hospital environment) to see
if a reaction occurs.

The results aren't always straightforward, so they should be
interpreted by an experienced doctor. (On page 191 I talk about
allergy tests that you can do online and why you should always
refer to a specialist.)

Elimination diets

Elimination diets are one way to explore whether a food allergy
is contributing to eczema flare-ups. They can be helpful in specific situations, but they are not a magic bullet in treating skin
conditions. Remember that food allergies are much less likely to
be a driver of eczema in adults.

Before undertaking any type of elimination diet, it is worth
keeping a trigger diary to see if there is any association between
eczema flares and foods eaten. This is fairly straightforward and
easy to do, as you just need to make a note of what you've eaten
for each meal and keep an eye on how your skin reacts. I would
recommend doing this for at least 2 weeks. Specific apps that can
help you to track your eczema symptoms and assess for possible
triggers also now exist (see Resources for details).

Elimination diets can help to identify trigger foods that are
responsible for causing delayed allergic reactions. As the name
implies, this type of diet involves eliminating a specific food
or group of foods from your diet for a period (4 weeks or less)
and then gradually reintroducing those foods carefully to see if
eczema flares. Although it sounds easy, it needs to be done with
caution, particularly if you are removing more than one food,

as it is important to maintain a nutritionally complete diet. I strongly recommend that you do this under the guidance of a dietitian or allergy specialist, as this process is complex and, in some situations, medical supervision is essential:

- Children: any child with suspected food allergies should be under the care of a medical practitioner such as an allergy specialist and dietitian.
- If you have a history of restrictive eating habits or disordered eating.
- If a 2-week diary reveals that there are several possible foods that could be causing allergies, you will need medical supervision to eliminate them and re-introduce them into your diet in a step-wise manner.

I do not recommend experimenting with cutting out foods/food groups yourself. I have mentioned before, but it bears repeating, unnecessarily eliminating foods from your diet that you aren't allergic to can *increase* the chance of developing an allergy to these foods later on.

Eliminating multiple food groups at a time can be problematic, without proper supervision, as in Inderjeet's case below.

CASE STUDY: THE DANGERS OF RESTRICTING FOODS

Inderjeet had not had an eczema flare-up for over 20 years. It wasn't until she was in her forties that she noticed itchy patches of dry flaky skin appearing on her stomach and arms during a period of significant stress. After several weeks, the patches started to spread and appear angrier, and although Inderjeet recognised that this was eczema, she was surprised that it had reappeared after many years. She thought that a food allergy had to be the cause and read about elimination diets online. She gradually cut out dairy, gluten, eggs, fish, nuts and seeds, and several fruits and vegetables. When she saw no improvement after several months of adjusting her diet, she finally booked an appointment at the clinic. Inderjeet couldn't understand why her skin had not cleared even though she had cut out all the foods that she suspected were causing her eczema.

Inderjeet had large areas of itchy, inflamed eczema with scratch marks over her body. She couldn't sleep and was struggling to work, as she felt so itchy and uncomfortable. I asked her about her diet and was shocked to hear that she was eating only a very limited number of foods each day, including brown rice and chickpeas, because she was too scared to touch anything else. She had lost two stone in weight and her eczema had not improved – in fact, it had worsened.

- **Step 1** Her blood tests showed that her iron and vitamin B12 levels were very low, most likely the result of the restrictive diet, so I prescribed supplements to replace these nutrients and gave advice on foods that contained them. I also referred her to a specialist dietitian to help support her and help her regain her lost weight.
- **Step 2** As stress had been a major trigger for Inderjeet, I suggested we find a mindfulness practice that would suit

her and we decided on a 10-minute guided meditation before bed.

- **Step 3** I recommended a gentle, restorative skincare routine including a new body wash and daily moisturiser.
- **Step 4** I prescribed specialist creams to manage Inderjeet's eczema.

Within 2 weeks her eczema was much better, and by 4 weeks it had completely cleared up. Thankfully, Inderjeet was able to successfully reintroduce the foods she had been restricting and her eczema remained under control.

Inderjeet's story might sound extreme, but it is just one of many I have encountered over the years. Although some people will require longer-term treatment for their eczema, an isolated flare-up can respond very well to prescription treatment. Early and effective treatment should be the aim. By delaying treatment, eczema can worsen, become infected and become even more challenging to manage.

Whereas food allergies certainly can play a role, unnecessarily restricting foods in an attempt to clear eczema (or any other skin condition, for that matter) can delay receiving medical treatment and can cause unnecessary distress. It can negatively impact your relationship with food and take the enjoyment out of mealtimes. We are increasingly aware of how restrictive habits can profoundly impact both mental and physical health.

Remember that a nutritious balanced diet is important for skin health, but unnecessary food restriction at the expense of our mental and physical health is not.

Red flags – unproven allergy tests

Search online and you can find a number of different 'allergy tests' that claim to be able to diagnose food allergies and intolerances. They are reasonably priced and widely available and promise to find the cause of skin rashes such as eczema. This can be really tempting, especially when you are struggling with your skin, but I urge you to avoid them. Examples include:

Hair analysis
IgG blood testing
Kinesiology (muscle testing)
Urine, stool or saliva tests
Vega testing

These tests are unproven, and there is little or no scientific rationale to back up their claims. IgG tests, for example, tell you about foods you have been exposed to and have recently eaten, not foods you are allergic to. I have mentioned before, but it bears repeating: restricting your diet without true allergies, particularly in children, can increase the chance of developing allergies to these foods when you try to re-introduce them later on.

What should I eat if I have eczema?

The SkinFood approach favours anti-inflammatory foods that will help support skin and gut health, which are two important aspects of supporting eczema-prone skin. As you have seen in Chapter 4, the approach can easily be adapted should you have specific food allergies.

Oily fish	If you can include oily fish twice a week, then do; it contains omega-3 essential fatty acids, which help form the protective skin barrier
Apples, broccoli and green tea	These foods contain quercetin, an antioxidant that helps to reduce histamine and inflammation
Probiotic foods	In early studies, imbalances in gut bacteria have been linked to eczema, and probiotic foods support beneficial bacteria. Try to include probiotic foods such as kefir, kimchi, sauerkraut or live yoghurt on a regular basis
Variety of plants >30 per week	Regularly eating a variety of plants is one of the best ways we can support gut health. Remember, as we learned in Chapter 3, this number can also include whole grains, oils, nuts, seeds and spices as well as coffee, tea, herbs and plain chocolate
Avocado	If you have a nut allergy, regularly introducing avocado or avocado oil to meals is a great way to boost your intake of healthy fats

Top five foods for combating eczema.

Eczema and supplements

A wide variety of supplements are marketed for eczema sufferers, but the evidence behind most is poor. In general, a balanced diet should provide all the nutrients you need, but Kayla's story below illustrates how nutritional supplements can be beneficial in treating eczema.

CASE STUDY: A LACK OF ESSENTIAL NUTRIENTS CAN WORSEN ECZEMA

Kayla had experienced eczema as a child and throughout adulthood, and it had persisted in a couple of places: behind her knees and in the crease of her elbows; however, in the year before she came to see me, Kayla had developed increasingly itchy patches that would not settle down despite using her usual moisturising creams.

When I met Kayla, she was frustrated. She had already undergone food allergy testing with an allergy specialist, but the results hadn't identified any dietary triggers. This is often the case in adults with eczema. As we spoke more about her general lifestyle and whether anything had changed in the past year, Kayla revealed that during the pandemic, she hadn't been able to go on her annual holiday in the sun. She also told me that she rarely ate oily fish and that her periods were quite heavy. I checked her blood tests for nutrient deficiencies and found that not only was she low on vitamin D, most likely from her lack of summer sun, but she also had low iron levels resulting from her heavy periods. In addition, she was lacking omega-3 in her diet. So, we turned to the 4-Step Skin Solution to offer Kayla relief from her eczema.

- **Step 1** We discussed how she could adjust her diet to incorporate foods rich in the nutrients that she was lacking, such as leafy green vegetables and flaxseeds. I also recommended specific supplements for vitamin D, omega-3 and iron, and we discussed how she might

improve her gut health by incorporating prebiotic and
probiotic foods into her diet.

- **Step 2** Kayla's eczema interfered with her sleep so we
  looked at ways she could improve her sleep quality,
  including applying her eczema moisturisers before
  bed as part of her wind-down routine and taking a low-
  dosage magnesium supplement at night.
- **Step 3** Kayla had struggled to find a moisturiser she liked
  so I recommended she opt for one containing ceramides
  to help restore her skin barrier.
- **Step 4** We addressed the inflamed patches of her
  eczema with prescription creams.

Following this routine, Kayla's eczema calmed down and
was nowhere near as troublesome as it once was. It has
now been 6 months since she first entered my clinic, and
Kayla's skin is not only nicely under control, but she's even
been making her own kefir!

Although supplements alone did not cure Kayla's eczema, optimising her nutrition alongside using prescription creams has
helped to keep her eczema under control. Here are some specific
recommendations for how supplements can help with eczema:

Vitamin D People with eczema can have low vitamin D levels
and this seems to contribute to more severe skin inflammation. If
you have eczema, it is important that you take vitamin D supplements through the winter months. If your levels are particularly
low, you may need higher strength supplements. (See page 85 for
details on dosing.)

Omega-3 It is worth considering supplements (500μg per day of DHA/EPA is required) daily if you are vegan, vegetarian or you don't eat oily fish.

Pollen food syndrome (PFS)

If you have hay fever and pollen allergy, you might have noticed itching, tingling or swelling in your mouth or throat when you eat certain raw fruits, vegetables or nuts. This reaction is typical of pollen food syndrome. In this type of reaction our body mistakes proteins in certain foods for pollen-triggering symptoms. I am personally familiar with this type of reaction as a hay fever sufferer myself, and I also notice my lips tingling whenever I eat kiwis and peaches.

It is very easy to mistake PFS for a food allergy, but the key thing to remember is that it doesn't usually lead to life-threatening reactions. Most cases are mild, but there are rare instances where it can become more concerning – if you're worried, make sure to speak to your doctor. Some of the most common foods that cause PFS are apples (raw), strawberries, kiwi fruit, Brazil nuts, almonds and walnuts. Other foods that might pose a problem include pears, peaches, apricots, melon, peanuts, carrots, cherries, nectarines, plums, oranges, celery and tomatoes.

If you've experienced a reaction to one of the foods listed above, don't feel that this means you need to cut out all of them. You should only consider removing something from your diet if you experience an uncomfortable reaction after eating *that specific food*. If you find that you're reacting to something that you love and don't want to stop eating it, you can try cooking (just a minute in the microwave is enough) or peeling the fruit or vegetable to reduce the intensity of the reaction; for example, I can eat cooked peaches without any issues, so test whether this works for you. An antihistamine tablet and drinking plenty of water also helps.

Reactions to foods that aren't food allergies

There are several other ways that our body can react to foods. These reactions are often confused with food allergies and can lead to quite a bit of worry and confusion, so I think it's important to set the record straight here.

Food intolerances

The terms 'food allergy' and 'intolerance' are often used interchangeably, but they mean very different things. Food intolerances describe a reaction to a food that, unlike true allergies, does not directly involve the immune system. Intolerances usually cause tummy symptoms such as bloating, pain or diarrhoea, but are not responsible for eczema flares.

A common example is lactose intolerance. People who lack the enzyme that digests lactose in milk and milk products can experience nausea, stomach cramps and even diarrhoea when they eat these foods. This is not a true allergy and instead is caused by lacking an enzyme in the gut needed to digest the components of milk.

Histamine in foods

I earlier discussed histamine with relation to rosacea. Histamine is a compound produced by cells in the immune system. It is important for many functions in the body, but when it is released in high quantities, it causes swelling and leads to itching. If you have an allergic reaction, huge amounts of histamine are produced by the body in an attempt to clear the trigger food from the body.

Certain foods contain their own histamine or promote histamine release in the body. This is not an allergic reaction, and these foods aren't a problem for everyone, but for some people with eczema they can worsen the symptoms of itching. One of the commonest culprits is alcohol. If this is something you are experiencing, remember that you are unlikely to be allergic to alcohol, it is simply because alcoholic drinks are often high in histamine.

High histamine foods include:

- Alcohol, particularly red wine. Gin, tequila and vodka are better options, as they contain lower histamine levels
- Aubergine
- Avocado
- Fermented foods such as sauerkraut and kefir
- Processed or smoked meats
- Spinach

I am often asked whether a low-histamine diet helps with eczema; this means eating only foods that contain low levels of histamines and excluding a number of fruits and vegetables. So far there isn't enough evidence to recommend it. Remember that histamine is a *symptom* of eczema and not the *cause* of it. This is also why antihistamine tablets do not cure eczema but can sometimes help with itching symptoms.

Key skin-friendly takeaways

1. For most people, eczema is not caused by a food allergy.

2. Food allergies can be divided into two types: immediate and delayed.

3. An allergy specialist can help to diagnose food allergies.

4. Delayed reactions are trickier to identify and may require a specific elimination diet under the supervision of a specialist dietitian.

5. Food intolerance testing is unproven and has no role in eczema.

STEP 2

The Mind—Skin Connection

CHAPTER 7

Nurturing Our Mind and Our Skin

Have your cheeks ever flushed bright red when you're feeling anxious or embarrassed, or do you often notice a pesky breakout before a big event? Our mind, emotions and the stress we experience can have a profound impact on our skin. Believe it or not, our mind is constantly communicating with our skin, influencing its function, behaviour and appearance on a microscopic level. This intricate relationship between mental health and skin health is known as the mind–skin connection, and I will show you why harnessing its power is an essential, but often forgotten, step in any skincare routine.

Stress and the skin – a two-way relationship

Our emotions play a hugely important role in many skin conditions; for example, about 80 per cent of people suffering from eczema and psoriasis report worsening symptoms when under pressure. After a particularly stressful day, you might wake up the next morning to find that you've developed dark circles, a washed-out, drawn complexion, and more visible fine lines and wrinkles. This isn't just all in your head; in fact, these are signs that your mind and skin are uniquely coupled.

It works both ways: not only can your mind and emotions influence your skin, but your skin can also have a profound effect on your thoughts and how you feel. Who hasn't felt a wave of embarrassment when a big pimple appears slap bang in the middle of your face? The visible nature of our skin means that it has the extraordinary power to influence how we feel. On a good skin day, we can be full of confidence and ready to run out the door without a single scrap of make-up. In contrast, there are other days where we feel an overwhelming sense of disappointment when we look in the mirror and just don't like what we see.

Almost everyone living with a skin condition will have experienced its impact on their mental health in one way or another. In the last decade, a new area of study devoted to the mind–skin connection blends the unique intersection of psychology and dermatology and is known as psychodermatology. Over the years I have been fortunate to work with leading experts in this field such as Professor Anthony Bewley and Dr Alia Ahmed. There are powerful stress-reduction tools that we can use to harness the power of the mind–skin connection and make it work *for* us rather than against us. These tools are essential, but they are often overlooked when it comes to caring for our skin, so whether you are dealing with acne or eczema, or you just want to improve how you feel about your skin, your mind is an important piece of the puzzle.

The Dermatology Life Quality Index

We know skin conditions can affect every single aspect of your life – from the clothes you wear to the relationships you have and even the job you take – which is why in 1994 dermatologists in Cardiff developed a new metric to quantify the impact of a skin condition on a person's life. Known as the Dermatology Life Quality Index (DLQI), this numerical scoring system starts at 0 (the least impact) and goes up to 30 (the most impact) and has been translated into over 110 languages and is used through the world.

It asks key questions about how skin conditions influence key areas of your life such as work, friendships and romantic relationships. Answers are then used to calculate a score out of a maximum of thirty points, with scores above ten suggesting that the skin condition has a very large effect on the person's life. In the clinic, my aim is to achieve a low DLQI score using the 4-Step Skin Solution to minimise the impact that skin complaints may have on a person's life. (You can try the test yourself, but please remember to share your scores with your care provider to help direct treatment. See Resources for the website.)

The stress response

How exactly does the mind influence our skin? The brain uses stress hormones (chemical messengers) to communicate with the skin. These are produced in response to any type of stress, whether physical or emotional, in order to prepare the body for perceived action. These mechanisms originally evolved to allow us to flee dangerous predators at a moment's notice, but the same processes still co-ordinate the stress response today.

When faced with a range of triggering scenarios – from the worry you might feel before a big presentation to the nervous anticipation you might experience getting ready to run a race, and everything in between – areas across the brain will fire stress signals. Such signals trigger the production of a cascade of stress hormones in a finely tuned manner. Think of it as an orchestra, with your brain as the conductor co-ordinating all the action. Cortisol is the primary stress hormone. We consider it to be nature's in-built alarm system, priming the body for imminent action.

The human stress response is so crucial that the body also has a second, faster way of responding to perceived danger. Stress signals in the brain also trigger the release of adrenaline, which causes an increased heart rate, raised blood pressure, and sweating and increased blood flow in the skin. It is this immediate rush of blood to the skin that is responsible for blushing. The point is that the body can't tell the difference between physical stress or an emotional stress, and it responds by producing stress hormones in the same way for both.

Charles Darwin once referred to blushing as 'the most peculiar and most human of all expressions'. If you blush, you will know exactly what it's like to feel the throbbing, burning flush rising in your cheeks when you feel worried, embarrassed or nervous. The redness that follows is there for all to see, and there's almost always a helpful someone who asks, 'Why have you gone so red?' Blushing is an example of how easily our emotions manifest themselves in our skin. Purely by thinking: *I'm embarrassed*, intense reddening can appear in a matter of seconds. The entire process, from worried thought to bright facial flush, takes only a few seconds. It is almost as if the skin is your second brain.

How does stress affect the skin?

Stress is an emotion that we have all encountered: it's that feeling of worry, anxiety or fear that keeps you up at night. Sometimes the cause is a specific event, such as a break-up or having to move home, or the stress can become more constant and lead to feelings of sadness and despair, culminating in depression. Anxiety develops when feelings of stress and worry persist, even after the original provocation has been resolved.

Almost all skin conditions can be worsened by stress. I can always tell when exam season is approaching, because my waiting room will be full of itchy teens with flare-ups of eczema. I've also known people whose psoriasis has flared up all over their body following a bereavement, but this doesn't mean that stress is causing the skin condition; it can, however, add fuel to the fire.

Stress and acne

You'll be familiar with this story: it's a big day, you wake up in the morning, check your reflection in the mirror and you're greeted with a huge pimple. The timing couldn't be worse, so you scramble to find a fast-action spot cream or you give in to impulse and squeeze. Research studies in students have demonstrated that increased stress is linked to more pronounced acne flare-ups.[1] This is because stress hormones cause sebaceous glands to turn the dial up on oil production and the excess sebum provokes inflammation, blocked pores and breakouts; however, there is so much we can do to break this cycle by combining the right skincare, mindfulness practices and prescription treatment, if needed.

Stress and skin ageing

The well-recognised features of skin ageing include fine lines and wrinkles, uneven pigmentation and loss of elasticity and firmness. I am sure that it comes as no surprise that stress can also impact how we age. I first described telomeres in Skin School on page 36; these structures protect the ends of DNA strands when cells divide, which is why they're often likened to the tips of shoelaces. Chronic psychological stress and raised adrenaline levels shorten telomeres, and the shorter they are, the more quickly a cell ages.[2] Persistently high levels of cortisol also break down collagen, which is the key structural component of the skin that's responsible for plumpness and smoothness. The combination of telomere shortening, collagen breakdown and chronic inflammation that stress causes can accelerate the skin ageing process.

Stress and rosacea

As we know, stress is one of the most common triggers for rosacea flares and can lead to flushing, redness and a burning sensation, but rosacea can also act as a source of stress and anxiety due to its visible nature. Studies have shown that people with rosacea may experience poorer sleep than those without.[3] This can create a vicious cycle as it's thought that a lack of sleep worsens inflammation, which in turn promotes rosacea flares. Getting a good night's sleep is so important for skin health so I'll share with you my key sleep tips later in this chapter to ensure that you're enjoying top-quality beauty sleep.

Stress and psoriasis

Studies have faithfully reproduced what I have observed in the clinic, namely that emotional distress can trigger flare-ups and worsen psoriasis episodes. Stress increases inflammation, as spiking levels of cortisol and adrenaline activate chemical messengers in the skin called cytokines. These cytokines activate inflammation and worsen skin rashes. There is a lot that we can do to help break this cycle with proven techniques, however, which I'll outline later in this chapter.

Stress and eczema

In people with eczema, the protective skin barrier doesn't work as it should, which means that skin can become dry, flaky and irritated. A recent study suggests that stress can actually stop our skin barrier from working properly and it might explain why eczema worsens at times of distress.

Researchers discovered that psychological stress in mice caused their skin barrier to weaken and become vulnerable to infection.[4] The stress hormone cortisol has been found to be responsible for these changes, as it causes the skin barrier to lose resilience resulting in dry skin. This directly worsens skin conditions such as eczema, where the skin barrier is already weakened, and it's likely that this also happens in humans too. In another study, medical students at the University of San Francisco were asked to fill in a questionnaire to report stress levels, and their skin barrier was then examined for permeability or leakiness.

The study showed that the students' skin barrier was weakened when they were under the highest psychological stress, such as during exams. Additionally, their skin barrier was stronger and more resilient when they were more relaxed and happier after returning from their holidays.[5]

Mind matters: the tools to tackle stress

Reducing stress can not only help your skin, but also make a profound difference in how you feel. You can tap into simple, effective techniques to promote calm and feel better from the inside out. In the clinic, stress-reduction tools are an indispensable part of the 4-Step Skin Solution, and Jeanette's case below illustrates why.

CASE STUDY: THE BENEFITS OF MEDITATION

Jeanette first developed eczema as a child, but now, in her thirties, it was getting worse. Her skin was so uncomfortable that she would be up most nights scratching it for relief. This went on for months, and she was fed up after trying all sorts of moisturising creams that did nothing to help alleviate her discomfort. When Jeanette turned up at the clinic to see me, she proffered a bag filled with all of the creams she was using (as many patients do). I asked her about her symptoms and when they flared up, and she responded that they'd worsened after a promotion at work. Jeanette's new role involved working longer hours with more responsibility, and she was exhausted. Her eczema was red and sore on her arms and legs, and her skin was dry. I knew that there were many factors at play here, and that the 4-Step Skin Solution would holistically address these.

- **Step 1** During our appointment, Jeanette explained that she didn't have much time for lunch so she would often resort to a cheese toasty and coffee. I explained how bringing more balance into her meals could help support her skin, and how she could use the easy principles of the SkinFood approach to help her to make nutritious choices. We looked at alternatives and she switched to bean soups with a wholegrain roll and olive oil for lunch, and snacked on nuts and fruit during the day.
- **Step 2** As stress was clearly an important trigger, I encouraged Jeanette to introduce a mindfulness meditation practice into her day, and explained how it would help to relieve her stress levels that were potentially causing her eczema to flare. We then talked about the best way to make the practice a new habit, which for Jeanette meant setting up a daily reminder on her phone.
- **Step 3** I recommended a soothing skincare routine that included a body wash and rich moisturising ointment.
- **Step 4** I also prescribed a topical ointment and explained how to use it safely.

When Jeanette came back to see me a few weeks later, her eczema had settled nicely and felt much less itchy – and

finally she could sleep again. The short, 10-minute guided
meditation that she had worked into her morning routine
had made a powerful impact on her overall well-being,
as it allowed her to start her day in a calmer and more
relaxed way. I have no doubt that this helped her eczema
recovery too. Although Jeanette came to the clinic about
her eczema, she took away a tool that would benefit her for
the rest of her life.

There are many ways to manage stress, and it is something very
personal. For some, exercise is a huge stress-reliever; for others,
a regular meditation practice provides calm, and, of course,
regular therapy, counselling and medical treatments can also be
hugely beneficial. The trick is to work out what works for you,
and this can be a practice that evolves and changes over time.

Mindfulness meditation

Practising mindfulness meditation will change your life. I could
end this part of the chapter here. This is truly one of the most
powerful tools we have to manage stress levels and boost positiv-
ity. You might think that it's strange to think about meditation
in relation to our skin, but there is now much scientific evidence
to back up the positive impact it can have on the mind–skin connection. And, from listening to my patients, I know that it helps.

Mindfulness meditation is an ancient practice that can be
traced back to branches of Hinduism from around 3,500 years
ago (1500BCE) that originally had its roots in yoga. Forms of
meditation are also thought to have evolved from Buddhism. It is
now a global phenomenon practised by millions, if not billions,
the world over. The word 'meditation' stems from the Latin word

meditatum meaning 'to ponder', and mindfulness is a practice that embodies present-moment awareness. It is a concept that can be tricky to digest, but in essence this type of meditation encourages you to focus intensely on what you are sensing and feeling in the moment without any interpretation or judgement. Any activity can evoke mindfulness; for example, walking, eating or gardening. Focusing entirely on the task at hand allows the quietening of your conscious mind and has a whole host of benefits.

My grandmother was devoted to her mindfulness practice. I remember as a child, finding it odd that she would spend an hour, two or three times a day in complete silence with her eyes closed. I had assumed that she was just taking a nap, as people in their eighties have every right to do; however, I soon learned that she was actually deep in silent meditation. She would often encourage me to give it a go myself, but as a teenager I couldn't think of anything worse than being stuck in my own angsty thoughts for 2 hours a day.

As an adult I came to meditation quite accidentally. A few years ago, I was incredibly stressed and close to burning out. I had worked long hours through each of my pregnancies, and I had three young children to look after, but then I took a job on the other side of London. The daily commute was over 2 hours. Combined with a pandemic, demanding hours and a hectic home life, I was exhausted! My sleep suffered and I started to feel anxious, but it wasn't until I discovered a podcast about the benefits of meditation that I gave the practice much thought. While listening to an episode I remembered my grandmother extolling its virtues and, although it had never really clicked for me, I decided to try a guided meditation on YouTube and began listening to it on the way to work each day. At first, the buzzing of the people around me was distracting, but after a few weeks I had trained myself to become fully immersed in a silent world and would awake feeling refreshed. As I opened my eyes, I felt revitalised, and I carried a pocket of calmness with me throughout the day.

Of course, I still get stressed, but I now feel that I can manage those feelings much more effectively. When I miss a few days or weeks of meditation, I feel it and then gravitate back to my daily practice without fail. A famous quote by one of the leading proponents of meditation, Dr Deepak Chopra, really rings true: 'If you're too busy to meditate once a day, you should be meditating twice a day.' By incorporating this simple step into your routine, you can enjoy life-changing results – and I say this from personal experience. Meditation gave me a new perspective, and I started to think about how it could also be harnessed as a tool to help my patients with skin conditions, so I undertook a week-long mindfulness meditation training course and learned more about the medical benefits of meditation.

Around 40 years ago Professor Jon Kabat-Zinn, a medical doctor, founded a contemporary form of 'modern-day mindfulness' at the University of Massachusetts Medical School. The revolutionary technique came to be known as 'mindfulness-based stress reduction' and he and his team conducted extensive research into the benefits of this approach in supporting a number of chronic diseases such as anxiety, depression, chronic pain and heart disease. In fact, one of the first conditions Kabat-Zinn studied was psoriasis, and he published this research in 1998.[6] The study involved two groups of patients with the condition who were undergoing treatment with medical light therapy: one group listened to a guided mindfulness-based stress-reduction tape during treatment while the other did not. The results were illuminating, as the group who had listened to the recording experienced significantly better skin improvements, and researchers were able to conclude that listening to the recording had reduced patients' stress levels, which in turn had produced a positive impact on their skin. The influence of the mind, our thoughts and our feelings on our skin can no longer be ignored. The British Association of Dermatologists has devoted an entire web page to mindfulness meditation that features five specific guided meditations for people living with skin conditions such as eczema and psoriasis (see Resources).

How meditation can help you

There are many benefits to mindfulness meditation, not only for your skin but also for your overall health and well-being. Here are just some of the things that it can help you with:

- Improve sleep quality
- Improve mood
- Reduce stress levels and the impact on skin
- Reduce social anxiety
- Reduce levels of anxiety and depression
- Improve your Dermatology Life Quality Index score (see page 203)
- Reduce blood pressure
- Improve concentration
- Develop a healthier relationship with yourself and better self-esteem

This is already a pretty extensive list, but there is even early research that suggests meditation can help to keep you younger for longer, because it is linked to having longer telomeres.[7]

Although more research is needed to confirm this, it makes sense given that emotional stress ages us.

There are many different ways to work mindfulness into your life; don't worry if you give it a go and it doesn't immediately feel right, because sometimes it takes a bit of trial and error to find a practice that suits you and your lifestyle. Spending 20 minutes of silent meditation might be the perfect way for you to start your day, whereas a friend might prefer taking a mindful walk in nature. There is no right or wrong way; the key is simply to get started.

Here are some of the most popular ways of introducing a mindfulness meditation practice, and hopefully one of them will resonate with you:

Guided meditations can be excellent tools for beginners, as they provide gentle instructions to help you focus your thoughts on your internal world. If you don't know where to start, I would recommend looking on YouTube, as there are lots of useful videos available, or you can download a mindfulness app. Here are some of my favourites that I used to get started:

Rising Higher Meditation, YouTube channel
Calm app
Headspace app
Chopra app
Insight Timer app
Happy not Perfect app
MyLife Meditation platform

The thought of consciously making meditation part of your routine might seem daunting at first, but remember that you can always start slowly with 1 minute mini routines before working your way up to a 15–20 minute daily practice – or even longer if you like. The great thing is that meditation is easy to incorporate into your day, as it can be performed anywhere, from a comfortable spot in your home (although not while you're in bed, as you are more likely to fall asleep) to your daily bus commute. As with any habit, picking a regular time and place helps to make it stick. I find often that mornings work best for me, but don't feel tied to do the same; go with whenever feels right for you. And finally, if you ever feel disheartened, remember that meditation is often compared to a muscle, so the more we use it the easier it becomes.

Basic meditation for beginners When we meditate, we are aiming for mindfulness: a present-moment awareness rather than the complete removal of all thoughts. The idea is to pay attention to your breath and take notice of when our attention wanders. Here's a mini practice that you can try:

1   Find a comfortable area to sit where you are well supported.
2   Focus on your breathing. A few gentle and slow deep breaths is a good way to start, before moving on to relaxed inhalation and exhalation.
3   Follow the pattern of your breath for 2 minutes. Try to notice whether it arises from your chest or your belly and the sensations in your body.
4   Continue for as long as you wish, gradually increasing the duration of each session.

Mindful walking This is one of my favourite ways to introduce mindfulness into your life. It incorporates fresh air, exercise and spending time in nature, all of which have added benefits for our well-being. Spending time outdoors and connecting with the world around us is incredibly beneficial, as it helps to boost energy, reduce stress, improve creativity and boost our mood. The traditional Japanese practice of *shinrin-yoku*, or forest bathing, encourages spending quiet time immersed in nature to promote a sense of calm.

Mindful walking is simply walking with present-moment awareness, so you pay attention to the lifting and falling of your feet, the sensations in your body as you walk, and the beauty of the nature that surrounds you. All you need is an outdoor space where you enjoy walking, and you're ready. My go-to spot is the woods near my house, but although I set out with the best intentions and try to incorporate mindful practices as I walk, sometimes my mental to-do list takes over. If this happens, don't beat yourself up, because just being outside is enough. When I look at the trees, the sky peeking through the leaves, and observe the abundance of new plants and birds, I know that regardless of how I felt when I started my walk, I'll feel good by the end of it. There is something so soothing about being in nature.

Journaling and the power of gratitude

Gratitude is a practice that is totally transformative. You might think that this sounds a bit out there, but bear with me. Being thankful and appreciative for what we have can set the tone for our day, as it helps to build a positive mindset. Neuroscience shows that gratitude contributes to our overall happiness too, lowering anxiety and depression, and boosting self-esteem in the short and long term.

Finding a space for gratitude in your day doesn't have to be complicated or time-consuming – it can be as simple as thinking of three things that you are grateful for when you wake up in the morning and writing them down. This practice is known as gratitude journaling. I keep a notebook and pen next to my bed for this very purpose, but you can always use a note on your phone to do the same job. There are some really lovely gratitude journals available too, which contain pre-filled prompts. On days when you don't feel good, reading back through your notes can put you in a more positive headspace.

In the clinic, I recommend journaling first thing in the morning, before you look in the mirror, as it helps to reframe the relationship you have with your skin. Try to choose one positive, compassionate comment about your skin or body. If you're struggling with where to start, here are just a few examples that can help:

- I am thankful that my skin is on a journey to healing.
- I am grateful that I am learning to take care of myself.
- I am grateful that my skin is protecting me.

(For more, have a look at the positive affirmation cards produced by the Real Skin Club. These encouraging notes are invaluable when rebuilding your skin confidence, see Resources.)

Remember that changing the relationship you have with your skin doesn't happen overnight, but these small steps can help to make the journey that little bit easier.

The sleep solution

Beauty sleep is real, and it's no surprise that sleep is one of nature's most powerful stress relievers. While we sleep, our skin cells renew and replenish, but it's also when our brain recuperates, which is why quality sleep is fundamental to feeling good.

Studies have shown that prolonged periods of poor sleep can accelerate skin ageing and lead to a weakened skin barrier too. One study even found that participants who slept better were perceived to be more attractive when compared with poor sleepers.[8]

So how much sleep do we really need? I recommend aiming for around 7 to 9 hours per night. Depending on your lifestyle this might seem like a lot, but I urge you to try prioritising your sleep – even if it's just for a week – to see how it makes you feel (and look!). There are many ways we can help to optimise our sleep so that we wake up feeling and looking refreshed.

Stress can interfere with your sleep, as the stress-response hormone cortisol, which I mentioned earlier, dampens the effect of melatonin, the key hormone that's responsible for controlling our sleep. The effect of cortisol means that we don't get enough deep sleep so we end up feeling fatigued and foggy in the morning. Melatonin also plays another important role as it stimulates the production of human growth hormone (HGH), a key player in skin health. HGH literally turns back the clock, promoting skin renewal, regeneration, collagen production and everything you need for radiant skin so it is no wonder that it is likened to the fountain of youth.

In addition to stress, certain skin conditions can interfere with sleep too: scratching at night is a common feature of eczema and psoriasis. The result is repeated night-time waking and difficulty getting back to sleep again. There are many proven ways in which we can improve the quality of our sleep, and here are some tips that I recommend in the clinic:

Maintain a regular bedtime routine Having a sleep ritual signals to our brain that it's time for sleep. It could be as simple as taking time over your evening skincare routine, a warm bath or reading a book. Just taking a few moments to wind down can make all the difference.

Engage in meditation A relaxing meditation routine (as explained on page 214) before bed can help to declutter your mind and allow you to doze off more easily.

Avoid mobile phone/computer screens This one is so hard to do, and it is something that I am really attempting to work on myself. Try not to look at screens in the hour before you plan to go to sleep, as the blue light emitted from digital devices interferes with melatonin and the sleep cycle. Despite popular belief, studies have shown that putting your devices on night mode doesn't improve sleep.

Avoid caffeinated drinks Caffeine has a half-life of 6 hours, which means that about half the caffeine in a beverage will be present in your body 6 hours later. Research shows that caffeine can alter the amount and quality of sleep we get. We all respond to caffeine differently, but if you struggle with sleep, try not to consume caffeine after midday.

Keep your refined sugar intake low Fluctuating sugar levels can also lead to poor sleep quality.

Keep your room cool and dark We sleep better at slightly cooler temperatures, and 18°C is thought to be the optimum. Use blackout curtains or blinds to prevent sunlight from disrupting sleep, as melatonin levels rise in darkness. Some people benefit from earplugs and an eye mask too.

Avoid strenuous workouts before bedtime Although exercise can improve sleep substantially, you should try to avoid it in the 2 hours before you plan to sleep, as the endorphin high can keep you awake.

Use pillow mists and sprays A quick spritz of a sleep spray really can help you to drift off more easily. Most of these sprays contain lavender oil, which can improve melatonin levels and aid sleep. I would, however, generally avoid these if you have sensitive skin or eczema, as essential oils can sometimes act as an irritant.

Try magnesium supplements You can apply magnesium to your skin in a cream or spray (transdermal magnesium) or take it as a tablet supplement. Whichever form you opt for, many people find it to be beneficial for improving sleep quality and duration. A dose of 250–300µg can be taken 1 hour before bed, although you should check with your doctor for medication interactions before starting.

Consider ashwagandha Known as *Withania somnifera*, ashwagandha is a medicinal herb that has long been used in Ayurvedic tradition for stress management and to improve sleep. Newer scientific research is now catching up with ancient knowledge, with several studies finding that regularly taking ashwagandha can help to reduce anxiety and improve sleep quality, including the length and depth of sleep.[9] If you struggle with sleep, you can try taking half a teaspoon of ashwagandha root powder daily, or 600μg taken in two doses. A delicious way to incorporate this is my Rose and Ashwagandha Beauty Sleep Latte on page 347.

As with all supplements there can be potential side effects, so if you're pregnant or breastfeeding, or have any underlying health conditions and are taking medication, please speak with your doctor first.

Additional tips for managing stress

There are also further factors to consider when trying to manage your stress levels to encourage happy, healthy skin – and we'll look at these now.

Exercise, stress and the skin

Regular physical exercise is a powerful tool to alleviate stress. Although there are the obvious physical benefits of exercise (including improved heart health and muscular tone), several studies have shown that it can help to calm symptoms of anxiety and depression. I usually recommend 30 minutes of exercise at least three times per week. This could be anything from a brisk walk to dancing around your living room to your favourite music. It really doesn't have to mean sweating it out in the gym for hours on end. Aim to incorporate some movement daily, and try to get outdoors if you can. It's so easy to get stuck at your desk all day, but a short walk and some fresh air can make a world of difference.

Yoga is an incredible practice that reinforces the mind–body connection. It brings together stress-relief, relaxation and spirituality in one activity. If you've never tried it, I would highly recommend giving it a go. I find this is the best exercise for recharging your batteries when you're running on empty.

Exercise releases the feel-good hormones: endorphins. You might have heard of the 'runner's high': that euphoric feeling you experience after sweating it out. This is the release of endorphins. As well as reducing stress, working out gets your heart pumping, improving blood circulation to the skin. This increased blood flow delivers additional oxygen and removes waste products, including free radicals. This helps to boost radiance and glow, naturally.

Not only is exercise important for managing stress, but regular exercise can also slow down the ageing process, ensure maintenance of muscle mass and support the immune system. Exercise is also anti-inflammatory, and it is thought that this is one of the ways that it keeps our skin cells younger too.

Exercise and rosacea

If you have rosacea, limit heavy, vigorous exercise if it worsens facial flushing. Instead, switch to shorter workout sessions or taking the intensity down a notch. Try to stay as cool as possible while exercising, either with a fan or air conditioning if you have it, and make sure to have a cold drink with you when you exercise – you can even use a cool spray or enjoy a cool shower to help your body cool down.

Food and stress: the brain–food connection

So far in this chapter we've looked at the unique relationship between the mind and the skin, but as we saw in Chapter 3 diet is also important for a healthy brain. What we eat profoundly influences our brain, including our mood and how we feel. There is a growing understanding of the role food and supplements play in the treatment of anxiety, depression, attention deficit hyperactivity disorder (ADHD) and many other mental health conditions.

A diet rich in fresh fruits and vegetables has been linked to increased happiness, better mental health and well-being, as well as a lower risk of depression. In a landmark study known as the SMILES trial,[10] participants with existing depression were introduced to a Mediterranean diet for 12 weeks. The results showed that simple dietary changes, such as increasing fruit, vegetables, oily fish and nuts, significantly improved symptoms of depression compared with medication alone. This doesn't mean that food replaces other available treatments, but that nutrition has added benefits for our brain and our mood.

Fortunately, the SkinFood approach described in this book has you covered. It turns out that the very same foods that we need for our skin also boost our brain. These include green leafy vegetables, oily fish rich in omega-3, antioxidant-rich berries and olive oil, nuts and seeds. In fact, you could say that SkinFood is also brain food. Following the SkinFood approach will not only support your skin health but healthy brain function too.

Skin therapy

Although all the practices mentioned so far are a great way to nurture the mind–skin connection, if you're still feeling uncomfortable in your own skin or you want to embrace a more positive way of thinking about your skin, you might want to try cognitive behavioural therapy (CBT) or habit reversal therapy.

Cognitive behavioural therapy

CBT is a form of group-based or one-to-one therapy. It's a technique used to address negative thoughts; for example, the stubborn voice in your head that tells you your skin just isn't good enough. There is good research that proves just how helpful CBT can be for many different skin conditions, particularly if you are experiencing low self-esteem and anxiety. Not only does it help how you feel, but studies have shown that it can even help improve skin conditions too.

It's so easy for negative self-talk to spiral. The purpose of CBT is to break this cycle, change thought patterns, and in doing so cultivate a more positive relationship with ourselves. When we think more positively, we can take actions that could actually help our skin and mood. If this all sounds a bit abstract, here's an example of how CBT helped Andrew with his thoughts around acne.

Andrew has experienced acne since his teens. He is now in university and his skin is having a huge impact on his social life. When his acne flares, he doesn't want to go out or see his friends, and he feels that his skin is holding him back from meeting someone.

Andrew's thoughts:

1 *I hate my acne.*
2 *I don't want to go out because my acne is so bad; everyone will stare at me.*
3 *I'll never find a partner because of my acne.*

Andrew's emotions and behaviours that resulted from these thoughts: he avoids going out and seeing his friends.

- He becomes anxious, frustrated and isolated.
- He gives up on his skincare routine or seeking help for treatment, because of an overwhelming feeling of 'what's the point?'.

Result:
Andrew experiences loneliness, anxiety and depression, and his acne doesn't improve.

In a CBT session, a therapist looks at each of these thoughts with Andrew, considering an alternative perspective to help to break hard-wired thoughts.

Here is an example of how the therapist would work through a negative thought:

Thought no. 2:
I don't want to go out because my acne is so bad; everyone will stare at me.

Reframing this thought:

1 What could be the alternatives? *I have acne, but so do many other people and they are going out.*
2 Do you really think everyone will stare? *Most people are too caught up in their own appearance to even notice.*
3 Is this a fair thought? *No, I am being really hard on myself.*
4 What would a friend say to you if you told them that this is what you thought? *They would say it isn't*

anywhere near as noticeable as I think it is and that I
shouldn't be avoiding people.

New thought:
Yes, I do have acne, but the reality is that most people are too
worried about their own appearance to ever notice. I can go out
and have fun; in fact, I deserve to.

New result:

1   Improved sense of self-worth.
2   Enjoyment and socialisation.
3   Greater likelihood of meeting a partner.

By challenging and reframing negative thoughts with more positive ones, not only do you start to feel better, but you are also more likely to take measures that can help your skin, such as sticking to a skincare routine or seeking help.

Habit reversal therapy

If you have an itchy skin condition, habit reversal can really help. Firstly, let's separate the terms 'itching' and 'scratching', which are so often used interchangeably:

Itching A sensation or a feeling experienced in the skin.
Scratching The action of rubbing the skin with your nails.

Sometimes we scratch because we're itchy, but it can develop into a habit that we do quite unconsciously. Ask yourself how often you're scratching because your skin actually feels itchy, and how often it's reflexive? There are other clues too: my patients who habitually scratch often report that friends and family frequently tell them to stop scratching, even when they don't realise that they are. Scratching is quite addictive, as it releases feel-good hormones that make us feel more relaxed, but unconscious scratching can damage the skin and interfere with the healing process, which results in skin conditions such as eczema persisting and becoming further irritated. This is known as the itch–scratch cycle.

Habit reversal therapy aims to intervene and break the cycle of unconscious scratching. It works very well alongside skincare and medical treatment (Steps 3 and 4). The first step is to create an awareness of unconscious or unintentional scratching, when it happens and what the triggers are. Once you have a level of awareness, it is easier to put strategies in place to distract or divert attention elsewhere. With time, this technique can be highly effective at breaking the habit of scratching and allowing the skin to heal. (See Resources for more about the mind–body connection from the National Eczema Society and Psychodermatology UK, as well as information on how to find a therapist.)

Seeking help

If you would like to explore either CBT or habit reversal therapy further, please do enlist the help of a clinical psychologist to support you. Remember that skin conditions can be accompanied by symptoms of depression or anxiety, or persistent low mood, so in such situations it is important that you speak to your doctor to see if any additional treatments might be helpful. I cannot stress enough that it is so important that you do not suffer in silence. Medical treatments can be life changing and life saving.

Key skin-friendly takeaways

1. The mind and skin are closely linked, and the mind can have a powerful influence over our skin health.

2. Stress management is integral for good skin health.

3. Mindfulness meditation is an effective tool for stress reduction.

4. Beauty sleep is real: aim to prioritise quality sleep.

5. Specific forms of therapy are available for skin concerns.

STEP 3

An Effective Skincare Routine

8

Nourishing Our Skin from the Outside in

It's late at night and you're scrolling through social media. You come across a post advertising a serum that promises to eliminate blackheads and leave you with smooth, poreless skin – and you're immediately sold. The only problem is that when you finally try this Holy Grail serum, it doesn't work in the way you expected and only aggravates your already sensitive skin. Sound familiar? Well, you're not alone. This is a story I hear time and time again.

Step 3 of the 4-Step Skin Solution is skincare, but not all products will be effective for your skin. Good skincare is all about excellent ingredients and finding the things that work for your skin type and concern. Having worked with some of the world's leading beauty brands over the years, I've learnt just how much research goes into making exceptional products; however, if a serum is designed for oilier skin and your skin is sensitive and prone to dryness, it's not going to be your friend, regardless of the quality of the ingredients. When you do manage to build a toolkit of skincare that works for you, it can feel almost magical.

The right products can have a marked effect on our appearance and our mental well-being, with our skincare routine acting as a form of self-care too. In this chapter I will explain how to build a simple and effective skincare routine as well as avoiding skin breakouts (acne) and how to keep your skin looking its best for longer.

Skincare in a nutshell

Now that we understand the importance of finding products that suit our skin, we are ready to identify our skin type and the products that would be the best match for our skin. To make things easier, have a look at the skin types below to find yours, and follow my tips on choosing the right products for you.

Dry/sensitive

- **Skin can feel tight after cleansing** Look for cream-based cleansers containing glycerin and ceramides to support the skin barrier.
- **Dry and flaky, especially in the winter** Choose rich moisturisers, which lock in moisture, and apply them to slightly damp skin for extra hydration.
- **Prone to sensitivity when using new products** Look for fragrance-free products, and avoid parabens, essential oils and physical exfoliants or scrubs. Be cautious with chemical exfoliation with AHA/BHAs, as they can disrupt the skin barrier further.

Redness

- **Tendency to flush or blush** Look for calming ingredients such as niacinamide and azelaic acid to help improve redness.
- **Sensitive skin that's prone to dryness** Go for a gentle hydrating cleanser and pat your skin dry after cleansing – never rub.
- **May have broken blood vessels on the skin surface** Look for green-tinted moisturisers to help minimise the appearance of redness.

Oily or acne prone

- **Pores may be enlarged in the centre of the face** Retinoids are excellent for keeping pores clear and can help to reduce their size too.
- **Prone to breakouts** Salicylic acid and gentle chemical exfoliants such as AHAs and BHAs in cleansers can help to prevent breakouts. Look for vitamin C to target pigmentation or redness after spots heal.
- **Skin becomes oily again soon after cleansing** Look for foaming gel cleansers and zinc sprays, which help mattify (reduce shine).

Pigmentation and uneven skin tone

- **Melasma, or uneven pigmentation** Vitamin C works well, particularly for deeper skin tones. Azelaic acid and retinol target pigment production and speed up cell turnover, resulting in a more even and radiant complexion.

- **Sunspots** Broad spectrum and a high-factor SPF all year round, and look for added iron oxide, as it helps protect against pigmentation.

Mature, perimenopausal or menopausal skin

- **Lack of hydration and radiance** Vitamin C and retinol are your two best friends for glow boosting.
- **Oily in some areas, dry in others** You can benefit from using different moisturisers on different parts of your face: lighter gels work for oily areas, richer creams for drier ones.
- **Acne affecting the chin area** Retinoids target breakouts as well as fine lines and wrinkles.

What skincare can do (and what it can't)

As much as I love skincare and skin products (and my own bathroom cabinet is a testament to this!), I also understand what they can and cannot deliver. They won't, for example, undo the impact that smoking, excessive alcohol and sun exposure can have on your skin. To understand why, let's take a look at how skincare works.

As I mentioned earlier, our skin barrier has evolved to be exactly that: a barrier repelling water and preventing the entry of harmful environmental toxins and bacteria. As it is so good at its job, it can also keep skincare ingredients out. The question is, how do we get creams that are applied to the surface of the skin past the skin barrier so that they can deliver the all-important ingredients to the deepest layers? Although some ingredients plump the outermost layer of skin (such as hyaluronic acid), the reality is that only a limited number of creams are effective at permeating the skin barrier.

NOTE Prescription skincare ingredients differ considerably from off-the-shelf products. They have been specifically formulated and rigorously tested to ensure that they work in the correct layers of the skin. Vitamin D creams used to treat psoriasis, retinoids for acne and wrinkles, and anti-inflammatory creams for eczema, are just a few such examples.

In terms of absorbing your skincare products, the size of an individual ingredient matters: the smaller the ingredient, the more easily it can penetrate the skin barrier, and the more effective it is likely to be. In the table below, I've outlined the molecular weight (known as daltons) of common skincare ingredients. Keep in mind that ingredients typically need to be less than 500 daltons in size to penetrate the skin barrier. The smaller the number, the easier it is for the ingredient to be absorbed.

Ingredient	Molecular weight (Da)
Salicylic acid	138
Vitamin C	175
Retinoic acid	300
Hyaluronic acid	5,000–20,000,000
Collagen (full length)	120,000

The molecular weight of common skincare ingredients in daltons (Da).

There are important exceptions. Some creams don't actually need to reach the deeper layers of the skin to produce results.

Take SPF for example, which largely sits on the surface of the skin, reflecting or absorbing harmful UV rays. You may be familiar with beta or alpha hydroxy acids such as glycolic or lactic acids. These work primarily on the skin barrier, and act as chemical exfoliants to weaken the 'glue' that holds the skin cells, allowing them to be sloughed off. The upshot is an instantaneously gratifying smoothed appearance.

Retinoids (vitamin A creams) are another exception. Retinol is something that I frequently recommend in the clinic. It is the gold standard anti-ageing and anti-acne skincare ingredient in dermatology as it's able to penetrate deeper layers of the skin through the hair follicle. Clinical studies have proven that it increases collagen and targets acne.

Understanding that there are limitations to skincare might come as a surprise, but it goes a long way to explaining why sometimes even the most expensive creams can be disappointing. If you understand how your skin functions, it will empower you to interpret skincare claims and assess whether or not they are plausible. My hope is that this advice will help to save you time and money.

What does a good skincare routine look like?

There really isn't a one-size-fits-all approach to skincare, because how our skin reacts to a product is completely individual. If you've got a routine that you're happy with, please don't feel pressurised to change it. I would, however, consider the following points when building a routine that suits you:

1   Cleanse your skin carefully morning and night by taking your time and massaging it gently. In the evening

you may wish to consider a double cleanse with either a micellar water or oil-based cleanser first to remove stubborn make-up or SPF. There is no need to spend excessively on a cleanser, as you'll be washing it off, so save your money instead for a moisturiser or serum that has a particular active ingredient that will address your skin concerns.

2   When it comes to exfoliators, I am really quite strict – *do not* use harsh scrubs containing beads and grains as these can damage the skin barrier and worsen skin sensitivity and dryness. Instead look for alpha or beta hydroxy acids to gently exfoliate and use these as often as your skin can tolerate. For extremely sensitive skin like mine, this may be once every two weeks, but if you're on the opposite end of the spectrum, you may find that exfoliating every other day works best.

3   Follow with a targeted serum that is tailored to your skin type; for example, serums containing hyaluronic acid will soothe dry skin, vitamin C will target pigmentation and improve radiance, and a retinoid will help to address signs of premature ageing.

4   Apply a moisturiser that contains ingredients to support your skin barrier. I recommend lighter lotions for oilier skin types and richer creams for drier skin. You can use an eye cream if you wish, but I don't think it is absolutely necessary.

5   Always use an SPF in the morning that suits your skin type and tone. There are many new formulations that blend seamlessly on all skin tones that can also act as a perfect base for make-up too.

Step inside the clinic: keeping acne at bay

Acne is one of the most common skin concerns that I see in the clinic, and there are some simple tweaks to your skincare routine that can help you to reduce breakouts and improve the appearance of scarring and pigmentation.

General skincare for acne

A consistent and effective skincare routine, combined with Steps 1 and 2, goes a long way to keeping acne in check. Start by assessing your skin type: is it oily-prone, drier, or is it a combination of both? Acne products are often developed to treat oily skin, but remember that not everyone with breakouts has oily skin. Some acne treatments can therefore be quite drying and not suitable for all skin types. Next, I'll explain these different treatments and how to incorporate them into your daily routine.

Cleansing

Starting with the basics, look for a gentle, soap-free cleanser that won't strip the skin's natural barrier. If your skin is oilier, a foaming cleanser is more suitable. If your skin is drier, a lotion or cream cleanser would suit you better. Remember to look for non-comedogenic products, as this means that the ingredients are much less likely to block pores and worsen breakouts. Some cleansers contain active ingredients such as salicylic acid or benzoyl peroxide, but, depending on your skin type, these can be a little drying. The other thing to keep in mind is that for these active ingredients to work they need to stay in contact with the skin. They won't work as well if you just do a quick rinse and run, so leave the cleanser on your face for a few minutes before rinsing it off.

In the morning, a single cleanse is sufficient; however, in the evenings, a double cleanse is required to remove SPF (which I assume you are, of course, using) and any make-up. Your first cleanse can be a simple micellar cleansing water (avoiding fragrance) applied to a cotton pad or a creamier cleanser massaged in well to remove all traces of grime. Please steer clear of oil-based cleansers, including natural oils such as coconut and almond, as these will only serve to block pores and worsen breakouts. Massage your cleanser for about 3–5 minutes for maximum benefits. Pat your skin dry with a soft, clean flannel and avoid rubbing.

Moisturising

If you have oily skin, don't skip moisturising, as this helps to regulate oil production. Oily skin can be dehydrated and flaky despite the presence of oil. Choose lightweight gel or cream formulations rather than heavy oils that can block pores. Excellent moisturising ingredients that don't block pores include hyaluronic acid and glycerin. It is easy to be tempted by harsh exfoliating scrubs in an attempt to clear acne, but these can actually make things worse in the long term by damaging the skin barrier and increasing overall sensitivity. If you have overdone it on scrubs and peels, don't worry – your skin will recover. Support its recovery with barrier-boosting ingredients, such as niacinamide and ceramides, and dial back on harsh exfoliants.

(Later in this chapter I will provide a morning and evening skincare routine schedule.)

Active ingredients for acne

There are active ingredients I reach for time and time again to help treat acne that have been proven to deliver results – although please do not use all of them in combination unless supervised, as they can lead to irritation in some cases. These ingredients work to target one or more of the four steps in acne formation, which are:

1   Increased sebum production
2   Blockage of pores
3   Inflammation
4   Overgrowth of bacteria

To make a plan for treating acne, it's important to work out what type of acne you have. We looked at each type in more detail in Skin School (Chapter 1). Certain ingredients are more helpful in addressing specific acne types; for example, if you have blackheads and whiteheads, retinoids and salicylic acid are fantastic and help to unclog pores. If your acne is more inflamed and sore, however, additional ingredients that can help include benzoyl peroxide and topical azelaic acid.

Over-the-counter vs prescription skincare

Skincare products that you can buy over the counter (OTC) can be very helpful for most people with acne; however, if breakouts are persistent or are leaving pigmentation or scars, prescription skincare products are recommended. We use higher percentages and more potent formulations in the clinic, although these come with a higher risk of irritation.

Ingredient	Benefits
Retinoids	Reduces inflammation, improves exfoliation to prevent blocked pores, reduces oil production, targets pigmentation (avoid during pregnancy). OTC and prescription forms available
Azelaic acid	Reduces inflammation, targets pigmentation and redness, reduces sebum production (available OTC or prescription depending on strength)
Niacinamide	Anti-inflammatory, reduces redness, restores the skin barrier
Benzoyl peroxide	Targets bacteria on the skin surface
Topical antibiotics	Targets bacteria on the skin surface and reduces inflammation (prescription only)
Salicylic acid/glycolic acid	Exfoliates the skin to unclog pores and also reduces inflammation

Ingredients that can be purchased or prescribed.

Retinoids for beginners

Retinoids are some of the most effective skincare ingredients for treating acne, and I love these for evening out skin tone, reducing congestion and preventing breakouts. They help to increase cell turnover, unclog pores, regulate oil production, reduce inflammation and tackle pigmentation and scarring. It's no wonder that retinoids are a Holy Grail skincare product.

Retinoids can vary greatly, though, and marketing can be deceptive. There are also many different forms of retinol, so in the table below I've summarised different retinoids, from entry level to professional prescription-only choices. More gentle retinoids take a few steps to be converted into active retinoids in the skin, which means that they cause less irritation but also tend to be less effective. At the other end of the spectrum, pro-level, prescription-only retinoids such as tretinoin can cause quite a bit of irritation, but the results do tend to be more impressive.

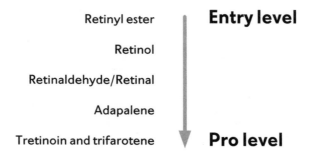

The varying strength levels of different kinds of retinoids.

Retinoids are notorious for causing skin irritation, so I always recommend introducing them carefully. How you respond to a retinoid varies from person to person, so start with more gentle retinoids and work up to stronger ones, depending on how your skin responds. Many skincare brands also have different percentages available, so start with lower percentages and move up to higher strengths as tolerated.

Tips for starting a retinoid

- Resist the urge for immediate results, and start by using retinoids twice a week to begin with, then gradually increase the frequency to alternate nights, and finally nightly.
- Use retinoids only at night, as this is when skin cells are most receptive to treatments – plus they can increase sun sensitivity which leads me on to . . .
- Use an SPF daily without fail.
- Use a moisturiser *before* applying retinoids, if you have sensitive skin.
- Avoid applying retinoids close to your eyes and mouth: these are trouble spots for irritation.
- You need less than you think: a pea-sized amount should be sufficient for your entire face.
- Scale back exfoliating acids in your skincare routine when starting retinoids, as they can contribute to further irritation. You can start to reintroduce them into your routine once your skin has become accustomed to the retinoid.
- It's OK to use retinoids a few times per week rather than nightly: they will still be effective, so go with whatever your skin can tolerate.
- You should avoid retinoids if you are pregnant, unless advised otherwise by your doctor.
- Be patient, as it takes time for retinoids to work. It can often take at least a few weeks to notice a real difference.

In the clinic I use prescription-strength retinoids: adapalene, tretinoin and trifarotene as the basis for any acne routine, unless someone is pregnant or trying to conceive. Not only do they target each step in the formation of a pimple, but they also help to tackle scarring and pigmentation too.

Azelaic acid

This is another of my go-to skincare ingredients. Not only is it anti-inflammatory, but it also helps to reduce hyperpigmentation and redness, and it is safe for use during pregnancy. You can buy skincare products containing azelaic acid over the counter, and we tend to use a 15–20 per cent concentration on prescription. I find that it helps to improve skin texture, brightness and redness by targeting stubborn pigmentation and post-inflammatory redness.

Salicylic acid

You'll find this ingredient in almost any pimple-fighting product. In strengths of up to 2 per cent it is anti-inflammatory and can penetrate the hair follicle to help unclog pores. It's able to target acne by reaching deeper blockages than other acids used on the surface of the skin.

Benzoyl peroxide

Benzoyl peroxide targets bacteria on the surface of the skin that contribute to inflamed breakouts. You'll often find it in leave-on treatments and washes. I particularly like benzoyl peroxide for targeting body acne, such as on the back or bottom. Cleanse with a 5–10 per cent benzoyl peroxide wash and leave on for a few minutes so that it can take effect. It can cause peeling and dryness, so go slowly, and be aware that it can bleach towels and pillowcases.

Skincare routine for treating acne

The following daily schedule incorporates cleansing, applying treatments and moisturising.

Morning:

1   Cleanse with a gentle cleanser for your skin type. You could use a product that contains benzoyl peroxide or salicylic acid, but leave it on for a few minutes to maximise the benefits.
2   Next apply an azelaic acid treatment. Allow 10–15 minutes for it to be absorbed.
3   Moisturise *and* apply SPF (non-comedogenic, of course).

Evening:

1   Double-cleanse to remove SPF and make-up using a suitable cleanser for your skin type.
2   Apply a thin layer of retinoid treatment.
3   Apply a targeted benzoyl peroxide or salicylic acid treatment on individual spots where necessary.
4   Allow the products to absorb for 10–15 minutes before applying a moisturiser.

This is an example routine and certainly not the *only* routine for acne, but it's a good place to start. You may have one that you prefer or has been recommended to you, and if that's working, by all means continue with it.

Make-up and acne

When you are buying make-up, make sure that you scan the packaging to ensure that the product is non-comedogenic so that it doesn't aggravate your skin. Careful removal of your make-up in the evening is also important, as its residue can block pores and worsen breakouts. The same rule applies to exercise: make sure to remove it before a workout, as the combination of sweat and make-up can be particularly troublesome for acne-prone skin.

Pimple patches

Tempted to pick a juicy spot? Try a pimple patch instead. It is so hard to resist the urge to pick and squeeze a spot, but please don't, squeezing can push inflammation deeper and result in scarring. Instead, take a warm shower and allow your pimple to come to a head. Apply a pimple patch overnight and this helps to gently draw out the contents of the pimple and reduce redness.

If Steps 1–3 have not been fully effective in keeping acne under control, head to Step 4 for additional medical treatments that will help to clear breakouts.

Radiant youthful skin

Who doesn't want healthy, glowing skin? It's easier to achieve than you think. Steps 1–3 of the 4-Step Skin Solution are your blueprint to radiant youthful skin. If you have more mature skin or there are specific outcomes you are looking for, that's where Step 4 (in-clinic treatments) comes into play. Remember, however, that treatments should be considered only in *addition* to a balanced, nutritious diet, stress management and a good skincare routine, rather than instead of. There is no point in trying to create the *illusion* of radiant youthful skin, because you really want to *live and breathe* it.

For clarity, the aim here is to protect and preserve our skin so that it remains healthy. We aren't trying to prevent every single line and wrinkle, as these are perfectly normal. I'm now in my forties and have started to notice wrinkles appearing on my forehead and around my eyes (lots of facial expression – what can I say!), and rather than fighting and despairing over these changes I'm trying to keep my skin healthy from the inside and out for the long term.

Sunscreens

We know that sunlight plays an important role in how our skin looks and feels. Uneven skin tone, premature signs of ageing and pigmentation can also be made worse by excess sun exposure. Although the effects of the sun don't appear immediately, the skin doesn't forget, and sun damage is something that accumulates gradually over time. Excessive sunbathing or sunburn also increases the risk of skin cancer in the longer term. From a financial point of view, it is far cheaper (and more effective) to regularly slather on the SPF than pay for costly cosmetic procedures later in life. The adage holds true: prevention really is better than cure.

We know that sunlight ages our skin, but why? Well, UV light reduces collagen levels in the deeper layers of the skin and, as we learned in Skin School, collagen is vital in keeping skin plump and youthful. Sunlight is made up of several types of rays, and the two most important to the skin are UVA and UVB. Studies have shown that UVA light causes collagen to be broken down and, when this happens, skin loses its elasticity and smoothness. You might think that you're safe during the winter months if there isn't much sun around, but UVA levels actually vary much less throughout the year than UVB levels. UVA can also pass through clouds and glass, so it's essential to use a year-round broad-spectrum high-factor (minimum SPF 30) sunscreen on a daily basis. (As explained on page 68, you will still obtain sufficient vitamin D with these sunscreens.)

If you have a deeper skin tone, SPF is still recommended. Even though pigmented skin has some in-built sun protection, this isn't enough to protect it from hyperpigmentation and uneven skin tone.

When it comes to picking a sunscreen, there is a huge amount of choice available. The exact formulation you select really comes down to personal preference, and I recommend trying a few options first to find the one that suits you best. The SPF number on the front of the bottle denotes how well you are protected against UVB and burning, while the phrase 'broad spectrum' (or four-plus stars) will ensure adequate UVA protection. For oily skin types I recommend looking for a non-comedogenic lightweight gel formulation, but if your skin is sensitive, mineral formulations containing titanium dioxide and zinc oxide will work best. For any concerns about hyperpigmentation or uneven skin tone, search for tinted sunscreens containing iron oxide that will provide additional protection against visible light (also known as blue light) as this is an aggravating factor.

How to protect against UV light

- Limit your time in the sun during the peak hours of 11am to 3pm.
- Cover up with a hat and clothing when you're outdoors in sunny weather.
- Apply adequate amounts of sunscreen – half a teaspoon for the face and neck is needed to achieve the rating on the package. Don't forget the back of your hands too.
- Apply sunscreen at least 30 minutes before leaving the house.
- Reapply sunscreen particularly after sweating or swimming.
- If your foundation or moisturiser includes SPF, think about adding a separate layer of sunscreen, as you will rarely use enough make-up or moisturiser to achieve the SPF rating on the package.
- Daily sunscreen not only helps with fine lines and wrinkles, but also uneven pigmentation, which can be a particular issue for darker skin tones.
- Sunscreen should be part of your daily routine, so to make it a regular habit apply it each morning after brushing your teeth.
- Consider taking a supplement containing polypodium leucotomos (see page 161) particularly in the summer months, when you're exposed to more UV light, as this can offer an additional protection from free-radical damage.

Skincare advice that works

In the clinic, I turn to research-backed skincare to help tackle signs of premature ageing and improve skin tone and texture. Skincare products don't have to break the bank, and there are many excellent cost-effective treatments. In addition to sunscreen, incorporating a simple but effective skincare routine is the next step in caring for your skin. At night, look for richer products to hydrate and support the skin barrier. We lose more moisture from the skin as we sleep, which is why heavier moisturisers are more suitable overnight. This helps the skin appear smoother when you wake up too.

A quick and easy routine could look like this:

Morning:

1   Cleansing in the morning with your cleanser of choice.
2   Apply an antioxidant vitamin C serum ideally containing ferulic acid to stabilise vitamin C.
3   Moisturise and apply SPF to the face, neck and back of the hands.

Evening:

1   Double-cleanse to remove SPF, pollution and make-up.
2   Apply retinoid product over the face and neck.
3   Apply a richer antioxidant moisturiser and eye cream, for example containing resveratrol

During a consultation, I ask a series of questions in addition to a skin examination to put together an appropriate skincare routine. The information I gather allows me to recommend a carefully curated list of ingredients for each individual patient. However, I can't offer tips on the exact formulation without meeting you in person, as this really depends on your skin type and preference. Below I've included a list of my favourite ingredients for glow. And they're my favourites for a reason: they deliver results.

Retinoids	Retinoids increase cell turnover, collagen production and combat pigmentation concerns, while also shrinking oil glands and helping the skin to appear smoother and more luminous. Read more about how to choose and use a retinoid on page 241
Vitamin C	Vitamin C is a powerful antioxidant with free-radical neutralising capabilities. It works well combined with sunscreen for additional protective benefits against UV light and pollution. Vitamin C can be found in many different forms, some more stable than others. L-ascorbic acid is an unstable form and needs to be formulated with other compounds such as ferulic acid to stabilise it so that it remains effective. I usually recommend 10–15 per cent concentration, but if you have sensitive skin, start at a lower percentage
Vitamin E	Another antioxidant, vitamin E helps to mop up free radicals caused by UV radiation. It also helps to retain moisture in the skin and can help with wound healing as well
Resveratrol	Found in the skin of grapes, this is an incredibly potent antioxidant with anti-inflammatory benefits. This is an excellent ingredient to look for in an eye cream, where using retinoids might be too irritating

Peptides	These are short chains of amino acids: the building blocks of all proteins. There are many different types of peptides available. When applied to the skin, they act as messengers, tricking cells into thinking that there has been an injury and to produce increased amounts of collagen in the skin. This results in firming and smoothing
Niacinamide	Niacinamide, or vitamin B3, helps to restore the barrier function of the skin. As our skin barrier can become weakened over time, this helps to rejuvenate it. It is also anti-inflammatory and therefore improves how well you can tolerate other skincare ingredients such as retinoids
Alpha and beta hydroxy acids	Hydroxy acids break down connections between skin surface cells and act as exfoliants. Care should be taken to avoid overuse, as they can compromise the skin barrier. They give a temporary improvement in smoothness and help to clear blackheads and breakouts. I find these chemical exfoliants are helpful when used once or twice per week to smooth and brighten
Hyaluronic acid	Hyaluronic acid is a natural component of the skin. When used in skincare, it draws in moisture from the environment to plump and soften. The result is that skin appears smoother and better hydrated. Take care to apply this to damp skin, otherwise it can dry your skin out

Some preferred ingredients for glowing skin.

Beyond skincare

Skincare isn't limited to the products we use and, in some cases, we can complement our skincare routine with at-home treatments. There aren't many great skin treatments that are free, but facial massage is one of them. Small studies have shown that regular facial massage improves the contours of the face and could even increase collagen levels in the skin, so it's definitely worth trying. You don't need to buy an expensive face roller or a *gua sha* to get going, just your hands will do. I find facial massage so relaxing, and I often do it for 10–20 minutes a couple of times a week while sitting in front of the TV. If you're unfamiliar with how it works, you can find lots of tutorials on YouTube.

There are also additional devices for at-home use such as microcurrent and LED (Light Emitting Diode). You'll find out more about these as well as more advanced treatments such as lasers and injectables in Chapter 9.

Skincare for rosacea

If you have rosacea, I'm sure you'll know that finding the right skincare routine can be a bit of a minefield, but in this section I'll break down which ingredients to look for and explain which ones target redness and which should be approached with caution.

Rosacea-prone skin is often sensitive, and a common concern is that skincare products sting or burn when they're applied. Look for a gentle, soap-free, alcohol-free and fragrance-free cleanser and moisturiser to avoid irritation. Try not to rub or scrub your face excessively; instead, pat it gently with a clean washcloth after cleansing. Overall, I recommend using fewer products and looking for minimal ingredients to avoid potential irritants. This means keeping your skincare routine simple: cleanse, moisturise/treatment and SPF should be all you need. The more steps you have in your routine, the greater the chance that products may interfere with one another and disturb the natural skin barrier, which we want to avoid, as supporting our skin barrier improves skin resilience. I also generally recommend being cautious with using acids such as alpha hydroxy acids and glycolic acids on rosacea-prone skin, as these can irritate. Retinols can be beneficial for rosacea but must be introduced slowly and carefully, starting with lower strength option first (see page 241 on how to pick a retinoid).

Here are some common ingredients that can irritate rosacea-prone skin, but remember that not all of these will necessarily apply to you: alcohol, camphor/menthol, anything scented, lactic and glycolic acid, sodium laurel sulphate and urea.

On the flip side, there are some fantastic ingredients that can help to soothe and calm rosacea-prone skin.

Ingredient	Benefits
Niacinamide	Look for formulations with up to 5 per cent to help boost and support the skin barrier and calm inflammation
Ceramides	This is an excellent ingredient in both cleansers and moisturisers that helps to replenish the skin barrier and prevent dryness
Azelaic acid	Formulations of up to 15 per cent azelaic acid are available over the counter, and it really helps to diminish redness and spots that can happen across the cheeks and chin. On prescription, up to 20 per cent azelaic acid is also available
Green tea	This powerful antioxidant can help to calm inflammation
Probiotics	Probiotics in skincare may also help to calm skin redness. These are interesting ingredients and the aim is to help normalise good bacteria on the skin surface, which can be out of balance in rosacea-prone skin

Metronidazole	The aim of metronidazole gel is to help balance the skin microbiome and reduce inflammation. It is particularly helpful for the red, bumpy type of rosacea
Ivermectin	This is a prescription skincare ingredient that we use in quantities of up to 1 per cent in a cream formulation. It specifically targets a mite called *demodex* that causes the red and bumpy type of rosacea
Brimonidine	This prescription ingredient can help to temporarily shrink visible blood vessels, making redness less obvious. It can be useful before a big event, but I don't recommend that it is used regularly as it can cause rebound redness when it wears off

Ingredients for calming rosacea-prone skin.

Skincare routine for rosacea

Here is a typical rosacea skincare routine that I recommend in the clinic:

Morning:

1 Cleanse with a gentle, skin-barrier-supporting cleanser and use tepid water rather than hot. Pat the skin dry after cleansing and do not rub.
2 Apply a serum containing any of the active ingredients in the table above and follow with a ceramide-rich moisturiser.
3 Apply a sheer mineral SPF; green-tinted versions can help to camouflage visible redness.

Evening:

1 Double-cleanse with a micellar water first to remove any make-up and SPF, followed by a skin barrier-supporting cleanser.
2 Apply a treatment cream/lotion (for example, one containing azelaic acid or a prescription skincare product).
3 Apply a calming moisturiser containing niacinamide and ceramides.

Simply introducing a supportive but targeted skincare routine can make a dramatic difference to rosacea-prone skin. Patience is the key: it takes around 1–2 months to see the benefits of a new skincare routine. If after introducing a new skincare routine, you're still looking for further improvements, there are additional treatments in the form of prescription tablets and lasers covered in Step 4.

Skincare for psoriasis

For most people living with psoriasis, it is likely that you will need to speak with your doctor to discuss treatment options, and often you will be offered prescription creams to help soothe the skin. A simple skincare routine, however, is also a must when it comes to psoriasis, as it will help to calm redness, ease scaling and soothe itching.

Skincare routine for psoriasis

Wash your skin with a gentle soap-free body wash and never scrub or pick at scales, because this will only serve to make the skin more inflamed in the long run. Next, use a fragrance-free moisturiser of your choice for comfort. Although a skincare routine alone is unlikely to clear psoriasis completely, it can help to reduce some of the symptoms.

In terms of additional treatments for psoriasis, including scalp psoriasis, the majority of these are found on prescription and you can read more about these, in addition to dermatologist-prescribed tablet and injection treatments for psoriasis in Step 4.

Skincare for eczema

Taking care of your skin is incredibly important if you have eczema. As the skin barrier is not working quite as well as it should, using a hydrating and protective skincare routine is essential. It's one of the best ways we can prevent and treat eczema flares. Even when your skin is calm and under control, don't skimp on your routine. When your skin barrier is supported and hydrated, it makes it much less likely for flare-ups to occur.

Start with a simple soap-free cleanser to wash the entire body. Have short showers with warm rather than hot water and avoid long baths, as they can dry out the skin. When you step out of the shower, apply moisturiser to slightly damp skin to lock in an additional layer of hydration. Take care to ensure that you are wiping the moisturiser away from the body in the direction of hair growth, as this will help to prevent blocked follicles. Moisturiser should be generously applied at least once a day, from head to toe. This could mean that you finish a 500g tub of moisturiser in a week, particularly if you are applying it more than once per day.

There are many ingredients I recommend looking for in moisturising and cleansing products, but here are just a few to start with:

Ceramides
Colloidal oatmeal (for adults without oat allergy)
Glycerin
Niacinamide
Petrolatum/liquid paraffin
Shea butter

These ingredients are proven to soothe, calm and help to restore the skin barrier. They are also highly unlikely to irritate or cause allergic reactions. It may take a few attempts to find a moisturiser that you enjoy using, but please do keep searching because the right one for you is the one you'll use every day.

A word on sensitive skin and skin allergies

If you have eczema, you may be particularly sensitive to products applied to the skin. Fragrances and preservatives commonly found in skincare products, such as body washes and make-up, can also aggravate eczema (for example, ethanol, sodium lauryl sulphate and lanolin). Even ingredients that are considered natural, such as essential oils and nut or seed oils, can irritate and cause flare-ups. In recent years we have seen an uptick in allergies to essential oils such as lavender oil, and fragrances such as Limonene and Linalool which are found commonly in creams for sensitive skin. It may seem rather counter-intuitive, and it often comes as a surprise to my patients, but this is a case where 'natural' isn't always better.

Ingredients in skincare can cause a few different types of reaction. One is an irritant reaction, where the ingredient causes the skin to be sore. The other is an allergic contact reaction, which is a true allergy to a substance that the skin has touched. Common causes of allergic contact dermatitis include fragrance, nickel, preservatives and hair dye. This type of allergy is much more common if you have eczema-prone skin. Skin can become even more itchy and inflamed as a result. We use a type of investigation called patch testing that helps to investigate such reactions.

In addition to skincare, there are numerous prescription treatments for eczema available, ranging from specialist ointments to cutting-edge tablets and injections. If this is something you think could benefit you, head to Step 4 to find out more.

Key skin-friendly takeaways

1. Skincare products enable us to care for our skin from the outside in.

2. Finding the right routine for you and your skin is personal, but it can make a huge difference.

3. A simple, effective skincare routine goes a long way towards keeping skin concerns at bay and preserving and promoting healthy, glowing skin.

4. There are excellent, targeted skincare ingredients that address acne and premature skin ageing or a loss of radiance.

5. Prescription creams are also available to clear stubborn breakouts, and there are many options to consider for long-term clearance.

STEP 4

Specialist Medical Treatments

9

Understanding Treatments for More Complex Skin Concerns

In the clinic, I recommend a 360-degree approach to skin health. This involves incorporating evidence-based nutrition and addressing the mind–skin connection in addition to skincare and more advanced treatments. These steps work in synergy with each other; it is not simply a case of choosing one over the others.

There are other additional measures to improve skin radiance, tackle visible signs of premature skin ageing and uneven skin tone and texture. Treatments such as lasers and chemical peels can vary markedly in price and effectiveness, but it's so easy to be lured in by clever marketing tricks that promise dramatic results. Spending more doesn't always equate to better results, as we have seen. Let's get into the variety of options you can explore for glowing skin.

Advanced medical treatments include prescription-only creams, tablets and injections. Choosing the right treatment is an individual decision made between you and your doctor. Included in this chapter is a summary guide to the many options available to alleviate the more persistent skin issues: acne, psoriasis, rosacea and eczema. In the clinic, I discuss the different options with each of my patients, and the decision made really depends on many factors, such as severity of skin condition, impact on life and convenience of treatment, to name but a few. You can find further details on each of these treatments on the British Skin Foundation and British Association of Dermatologists websites (see Resources).

In-clinic facials and treatments

There is such an enormous array of in-clinic or in-spa facials available that I couldn't possibly cover each and every one. Here are some of the most popular treatments that address specific concerns.

Chemical peels

Chemical peels use acids, such as lactic acids or glycolic acids, at percentages that dissolve the outermost layers of the skin. Different peels have varying purposes depending on their ingredients. Some are better for pigmentation whereas others are effective for fine lines.

I think that gentle chemical peels can be helpful for rejuvenation and clearer skin but, a word of warning: results may be short-lived. The skin barrier will eventually build back up again, as it is meant to do. Overzealous peels can irritate and worsen pigmentation, so be sure to seek out an experienced practitioner.

LED Light

LED (light-based) therapies deliver focused light energy waves to the skin for a variety of purposes. LED treatments come in a range of different colours, each with differing beneficial properties. Red-light treatments promote the skin's natural heal-ing mechanisms, which helps to improve radiance, calm redness and soften the appearance of fine lines by increasing collagen in the skin. Blue-light wavelengths are anti-bacterial and most suited to acne-prone skin, while green-light offers benefits for hyperpigmentation and uneven skin tone. You can obtain LED mask devices for home use; some of these can be effective, but you have to use them consistently to see results. In-clinic treat-ments are more effective, as they deliver higher-strength doses of specific wavelengths of light.

Laser treatments

Laser devices shine bright energy waves to improve the appear-ance of the skin. There are a myriad of lasers on offer and their numbers are increasing rapidly. Each type of laser can address a different skin concern, with some better for pigmentation, some for wrinkles and others for skin tightening. There are also powerful lasers (such as CO_2) that can provide dramatic results to improve the appearance of acne scarring. Lasers work very differently on each skin tone and for each concern, so it is important to seek out an experienced practitioner.

Microneedling

This is another popular technique that uses a device to roll tiny needles into the upper layers of the skin. It's offered in many beauty spas, and there are even at-home devices available. I would recommend going to a dermatology clinic or experi-enced aesthetic practitioner to receive microneedling treatment, because unless the little needles penetrate into the dermis, where collagen is produced, it is unlikely to be all that beneficial.

Radiofrequency microneedling is a more advanced version of

traditional microneedling. This procedure delivers heat energy through the microneedling device to the dermis to promote new collagen production, resulting in tighter, rejuvenated skin. This can help with both sagging skin and scarring. Although it works well, it can be painful!

Microcurrent

Microcurrent devices deliver a tiny dose of electrical currents to muscles in the face and the skin cells. It works to tighten and tone facial muscles for a lifted appearance. As with many of these treatments, there are devices that you can use at home or you can experience microcurrent treatment at a clinic. I am a fan of microcurrent, as it is entirely non-invasive and delivers very natural results. If you opt for a home device, any improvement is entirely dependent on how consistently you use it.

Cosmetic treatments – my advice

I'm sure I've made it fairly clear by now that cosmetic procedures should always be seen as added extras and the very last step in skincare. There really is no point in spending hundreds of pounds (or more) for these treatments if you aren't looking at Steps 1–3 first. This is as futile as using mouthwash but not brushing your teeth! Many of these treatments offer a quick fix and temporarily smooth skin, which can be so alluring. But remember that long lasting improvements in your skin (and your health) come from the habits you adopt every day: nutrition, mindfulness, quality sleep and an effective skincare routine with daily sunscreen.

There is no doubt that carefully placed cosmetic fillers can give natural results to restore facial contours. Judicious use of botulinum toxin (botox) can also help to prevent lines and wrinkles by limiting repeated muscle movement. Recently developed 'skin boosters' also deliver a range of vitamins into the dermis to promote collagen production, although I would always prefer to get these vitamins from the diet.

I am concerned, though, by the growing number of younger and younger patients requesting cosmetic treatments, as they are not without potential complications. The rising trend is attributed to the immeasurable influence of social media, with both 'filler face' and 'filter face' becoming increasingly common. It is almost impossible to achieve in real life what is presented online in filtered and Photoshopped images, and in attempting to do so you could jeopardise your health as well as your finances.

Exposure to heavily airbrushed images can contribute to feelings of low self-worth and dysmorphia – a medical condition where you develop obsessive negative thoughts about your own appearance. If this is all sounding a little too familiar, make sure to consult your doctor, as there is help available.

The success of any procedure really does depend on the practitioner delivering it. Correctly placed botox and filler can look natural and restorative, whereas incorrect placement can result in an artificial, frozen or puffy look. This is one area where experience, expertise and an artful eye really do matter, so be very wary of misleading claims.

My advice is to think very carefully before you commit to any procedures, and be sure to research the clinic and practitioner you're considering. I would always recommend seeking out an appropriately qualified medical practitioner such as a dermatologist, cosmetic doctor, plastic surgeon or specialist nurse who has undergone the necessary training. Not only should the practitioner be able to deliver the treatment with expertise and experience, but more importantly, they should also be able to manage any potential complications promptly. (See Resources for a link to find certified practitioners.)

Additional treatment options for more complex skin concerns

If you've tried Steps 1–3 of the 4-Step Skin Solution, but still feel that your skin needs more attention, then you might want to consider additional treatment options such as over-the-counter products or prescribed medication. We'll now look at what treatments you might consider for the most common skin concerns that I see in the clinic.

Medical treatments for acne

In the clinic, we offer both prescription skincare and tablets to treat acne, so it's important that you are familiar with the different options so that you and your doctor can decide on which ones to try.

Specific antibiotics can be used to treat acne, and these are taken for several months at a time. The most frequently used are lymecycline and doxycycline. As we covered in Chapter 3, I often recommend a probiotic that helps to protect gut bacteria while on long-term antibiotic treatment, and it can also help ameliorate side effects such as bloating or diarrhoea.

Another option is a prescription-only tablet called isotretinoin, which is derived from vitamin A and commonly known as Roaccutane. Although for some people it can offer a permanent solution to acne, there are some very important things to consider before you start taking it; for example, it might not be for you if you suffer from depression or anxiety, as isotretinoin has been linked to changes in mood. You would also need to ensure that you are on effective contraception if you could potentially become pregnant during treatment, as it's extremely harmful to unborn babies. Due to these potential side effects, isotretinoin can only be prescribed in the UK under the supervision of a consultant dermatologist. Some patients may experience dry skin and eyes during treatment, as well as high cholesterol. In the clinic, I often recommend omega-3 supplements are taken at a dose of 500μg DHA/EPA daily to help with some of these symptoms of dryness.

If you experience hormonal acne and/or polycystic ovarian syndrome (PCOS), with breakouts worsening before your menstrual cycle, there are also other treatment options to consider. There are types of combined oral contraceptive pill (such as Yasmin) that can benefit hormonal acne. Spironolactone is another tablet we use to treat hormonal acne, and it works by lowering the impact of androgen hormones on the skin – again, this is not a suitable medication to take when pregnant. Spironolactone is also useful in the treatment of perimenopausal and menopausal acne and does not interfere with hormone replacement therapy.

For some people targeted blue LED treatments are also helpful, as this particular wavelength of light targets bacteria on the skin and reduces inflammation. Blue light can be delivered in the clinic or at home in the form of light-therapy masks. The latter tend to be less effective and require consistent use to see results. I find blue light can be useful for patients who do not wish to take tablets but haven't achieved their desired results with Steps 1–3.

One caveat to light therapy is that it tends to work only when you are using it, and acne can reappear when you stop.

If you have a big occasion coming up or a persistent individual acne cyst, this can also be injected with a tiny amount of steroid to reduce pain and swelling. Chemical peels can also be used for mild to moderate acne and will temporarily improve the appearance of the skin, making it appear smoother and decongesting pores. Regular treatments are often required to maintain results.

As always, the decision as to which treatment to go for should result from a joint discussion between you and your doctor.

Medical treatments for rosacea

In the clinic, in addition to Steps 1–3, I also use a combination of prescription creams or tablets to treat persistent rosacea, or you can try light treatments and specific lasers. The type of approach you opt for is a very personal decision that also depends on the type of rosacea you have. Tablets for rosacea tend to be more helpful for the bumpy/spotty sub-type known as papulopustular rosacea. We use low doses of antibiotic tablets such as doxycycline or lymecycline taken for several weeks or months at a time, and this helps to calm redness and reduce spots. Some patients may be concerned about the effects of taking antibiotics for prolonged periods of time on gut bacteria, but these are usually prescribed in quite low doses. In addition, I always recommend taking a good quality probiotic alongside antibiotics to protect gut bacteria (see page 92 for advice on choosing a probiotic).

For stubborn rosacea, we can also use a tablet medication called isotretinoin, derived from vitamin A, at a very low dose. It isn't suitable for everyone (as I explained on page 268), but it can be taken for a longer period of time to help diminish redness and reduce bumps and spots on the skin.

If your primary concern is stubborn redness, rather than spots, lasers and light treatments are highly effective. You can try at-home red LED therapy masks which can control redness symptoms. As I have mentioned earlier, these devices need to be used consistently to achieve results – just pop your mask on and multi-task with a meditation in the evening. If you struggle with more persistent redness or want to achieve improvements quickly then in-clinic treatments are more likely to help. The most frequently used types are pulse-dye laser and intense pulsed light. These lasers target blood vessels near the surface of the skin and can also help to calm inflammation. Often a series of treatments is needed to deliver results, although some people can see an improvement after a single treatment. Please do seek out an experienced specialist to discuss the right treatment option for you. If you have a deeper skin tone, there are specific lasers suitable, and an experienced practitioner will be able to guide you. Using the wrong type of laser on deeper skin tones can result in burning and pigmentation. (If you are looking for a laser provider, have a look at the register on the Joint Council of Cosmetic Practitioners website, see Resources.)

Medical treatments for psoriasis

Before we discuss treatment, let's consider psoriasis severity:

- **Mild** involves under 3 per cent of the body, including areas such as the scalp, elbows and knees.
- **Moderate** involves 3–10 per cent of the body, including

additional areas such as the torso.

- **Severe** involves over 10 per cent of the body, including large areas of the skin. If your psoriasis involves visible areas of the body, such as the face or chest, it is also considered to be severe.

In addition to the physical effect of the skin condition, we also consider the impact on mental health and well-being. To do this we use the Dermatology Life Quality Index (page 203). More severe psoriasis or cases that have a greater impact on mental health are more likely to require hospital-based treatments.

Your doctor will be able to recommend prescription treatments for the affected skin and this often includes vitamin D creams that may also contain anti-inflammatory steroids. These treatments come in different formulations; for example, ointments, creams or even sprays. Follow the instructions carefully so that you use the correct amount for the appropriate duration. Other anti-inflammatory creams are available without steroids, and these are more suitable for the face. Such creams contain the ingredients pimecrolimus or tacrolimus, which work to calm inflammation in the skin.

If you have scalp psoriasis, use a medicated shampoo such as one containing coal tar. This can be purchased without a prescription. These shampoos help to lift off scales and reduce itching and inflammation. There are further specific treatments for the scalp, including lotions and ointments, which are also available on prescription. (In the clinic I point patients to an excellent video on how to treat psoriasis in the scalp from the team at Guy's and St Thomas' NHS Trust, see Resources.)

If prescription creams are not helping, and your psoriasis is more extensive or impacting your quality of life, the next step to consider is dermatological treatments. You would need to speak with your GP, who can refer you to a dermatology clinic to discuss which treatment would best suit you. Much of my work in the NHS has revolved around assessing people with severe psoriasis and guiding them towards an appropriate treatment, so I'll share some of the options that might be offered to you.

Phototherapy

Medical light therapy (phototherapy) is a helpful treatment for psoriasis, particularly if your skin improves in the sun naturally. It involves standing in a medical light booth that emits a small part of the UVB light spectrum, two or three times per week. These are very different from sunbeds, which are not regulated and dramatically increase the risk of skin cancer.

It takes about twenty to thirty sessions in a medical light booth to improve the skin, but for some people it can be highly effective. The upside of the treatment is that no tablets are required and there are few side effects, although for some people this is not a suitable treatment; for example, if they are at high risk of sunburn or skin cancer.

Tablets and injections

If you have more persistent psoriasis that covers wider areas of skin or you also experience joint inflammation, known as psoriatic arthritis, it may be necessary to use tablets or injection treatments. These therapies work to clear the skin by targeting the immune system, which often goes into overdrive in cases of psoriasis. Tablets include acitretin, methotrexate and cyclosporine and they work by reducing underlying inflammation.

We now have a much better understanding of the inflammation that drives psoriasis, and there has been a revolution of new treatments specifically designed to target the driving causes. Remarkably, many of these treatments allow patients to experience clear skin for the first time. It is truly life changing, as we'll now see in Sanjeev's case.

CASE STUDY: LIFE-CHANGING TREATMENT

Sanjeev had experienced psoriasis since childhood. It had an enormous impact on his life, and he had lost confidence throughout his teens as a result of the red, scaly rash on his body. He was bullied at school, but he worked hard to go to university and landed a job in marketing after graduation. When I met Sanjeev for the first time, he was taking prescription tablets for his skin. Despite changing his diet and lifestyle, and taking his medication regularly, his skin was about 15 per cent covered in psoriasis and it was clear that his medication was not working. We talked about a type of injection treatment for psoriasis called a biologic. Given the severity of his skin and the impact on his life, Sanjeev would qualify for this treatment under the NHS.

Within 3 months of commencing this new treatment, Sanjeev returned to my clinic ecstatic. His skin was clearing, and it was in better shape than it had ever been. After 6 months, Sanjeev came to the clinic with his new girlfriend. He had never had the confidence before to date, but he now felt that he had his life back. He brought with him his family photograph album for me to look at, and I flicked through. Surprisingly I could not find a single photo of Sanjeev. He shared that, since he was a child, he had refused to have his photo taken because he was so embarrassed about his skin. When I heard this, it took everything not to burst into tears. Sanjeev was a new man, which was so rewarding to see.

Sanjeev's life was transformed with a new treatment, and it's possible for anyone else living with psoriasis too. If prescription tablets aren't working for you, speak with your dermatologist to see if there are other options you can try. There are so many new approaches available that there is no reason to suffer with psoriasis. For further information on these treatments, please see the Psoriasis Association and British Association of Dermatologists websites (see Resources).

Medical treatments for eczema

Skincare is a critical step in keeping eczema flares under control; however, when it is no longer effective on its own, prescription creams, tablets and injections are also available to settle irritated, inflamed skin. As eczema flares can hinder sleep, work and social activities, it's important to address them early on.

We use prescription creams to treat troublesome eczema. There are different types and strengths of creams and ointments, which include steroid and non-steroid treatment creams to help manage eczema flares. We generally recommend using these to clean dry skin and waiting 10 minutes before applying moisturiser. It is important to follow instructions from your healthcare provider carefully on the following:

- How much to apply and how often.
- Which areas of the body to use specific creams on (there will usually be different options for the face and body).
- How long to use them for.
- What to do if the creams don't help.

For many, using prescription skincare is a safe and effective way to help keep eczema under control. I have seen some patients who have had concerns about using steroid creams, but these can be used safely with clear, careful instructions. If this is something that concerns you, speak with your doctor. There are other treatment options available such as non-steroid creams that contain inflammation-calming ingredients such as pimecrolimus and tacrolimus.

If eczema is having a significant effect on your quality of life and you've already tried applying prescription skincare, it might be time to consider other options.

Phototherapy

Medical light therapy (phototherapy), as mentioned above for psoriasis, is suitable for some types of eczema, particularly if your eczema improves in the summer months. You need to attend a clinic regularly for treatment, often two or three times per week, and a course of around twenty to thirty treatments is needed to see benefits.

Tablets and injections

Fortunately, there are now several tablet treatments available for eczema. These include steroid tablets (as mentioned on page 273), methotrexate and cyclosporine among others. All these treatments work to calm the overactive immune response that drives eczema inflammation. In doing so, such treatments reduce redness, scaling and itching. These are medications I have been prescribing in the NHS for many years and they can be highly effective, but you need to find the right one for you.

For some, these treatments are required for short periods of time to settle a flare, whereas for those with more longstanding eczema they are used for months or years at a time. If such treatments are not appropriate or they are ineffective, you may be eligible for newer treatments for eczema. These include an injection (dupilumab) or a newer type of tablet (JAK inhibitor). I work in a specialist NHS clinic to prescribe such treatments, and although they can be incredibly beneficial, they are not without possible side effects that need to be carefully considered. (Excellent information is available on each of these topics on the National Eczema Society and British Association of Dermatologists websites, see Resources.)

Whatever skin concern you may have, my aim is to illustrate just how many different possible options there are. I want you to feel empowered in the knowledge that you can address your skin concern, whatever it may be, from both the inside *and* the outside.

Key skin-friendly takeaways

1. Step 4 looks at prescription skincare and medical treatments for a range of common skin concerns. Think of these steps (and those in Step 3) *in addition* to, rather than instead of Steps 1 and 2; remember that all four steps work together in synergy to maximise results.

2. Anti-ageing treatments and cosmetic procedures have their place, but make sure to seek out an experienced, registered practitioner.

3. Prescription creams offer a more potent treatment option for more persistent skin concerns.

4. Remember to speak with a doctor about treatment options, if you feel that your skin condition is beginning to impact your quality of life. How your skin makes you feel matters just as much as how it looks.

5. There are highly effective medical treatments such as light therapy, tablets or injections to address skin conditions such as acne, eczema, rosacea and psoriasis – there really is no need to suffer.

10

Eat to GLOW: SkinFood in the Kitchen

It's now time to put everything we've learned so far into practice, and to do this I'll share with you some of my favourite nutritious and flavoursome recipes. I love to cook and experiment with new recipes, but as a busy working mum of three I simply don't have that much time to spend in the kitchen. For me, meals need to be quick, tasty, and to combine the key elements of GLOW (greens, lean protein, oils and healthy fats, and whole grains). Some of the recipes included here are merely an assembly job, and all ingredients should be available in supermarkets. In Chapter 4 we discovered why 'eating the rainbow' is one way to achieve radiant skin. In the following pages you'll find bright, vibrant recipes that taste as good as they look.

The key to introducing any changes to the way you eat is preparation, and many psychologists explain that mental preparedness is the very first step towards any form of change in your behaviour. One way to think about it is using the 'why, how, what method' devised by Simon Sinek in his book *Start with Why*. I recommend that you make a few notes either in a notebook or on your phone to answer the following questions:

1 First, think about *why* you want to make changes What will the impact be on your long-term health and well-being? Are you spending too much on takeaways or ready meals? Are you eating the same meals day after day? Think about how you want to feel when you make changes to your diet.

2 Next, think about *how* you will make these changes How can you adjust your day-to-day eating habits to incorporate the GLOW principles of the SkinFood approach? Start by considering what you usually eat over the course of a week: what are your favourite meals; how can these be tweaked to optimise nutrients?

For example, if you start the day with toast and jam, you could swap white bread for wholegrain, top your toast with almond butter for protein and healthy fats, and finish with a side of fruit. If you love pasta and meatballs, you can use the same principle and switch to wholegrain pasta, add some extra veggies to your sauce and use lean turkey, chicken mince or even lentils instead of beef.

3 Now consider *what* you need to do to create an environment that supports the changes you want to make – in other words how can you make it easy to follow the SkinFood approach? Have a look through the recipes on the following pages and see which ones you'd like to try. Note down any ingredients you need according to your budget, and then check your fridge, freezer and storecupboard to see what you might already have to hand. Think about snacks too, and try to make sure you have plenty of healthy choices – I take an apple and a small handful of cashew nuts to work with me most days in my bag to stave off hunger pangs. It's a quick and easy snack that takes no time to prepare, which is perfect for when I'm rushing out the door in the morning.

4 Finally, *be kind* to yourself Remember that the SkinFood approach is not a restrictive diet; enjoy the foods you love – and that includes a scoop of ice cream, some pizza or French fries now and again. Just be mindful of your overall balance: if most of your meals are nutritious, there is of course room for these little pleasures.

In the clinic, I don't recommend a regimented meal plan, instead I work on adjusting the existing structure of my patients' diets to boost nutrients and flavour, so that not only do they enjoy their meals, but they feel good too.

My top ten SkinFoods

These are the top foods that I recommend you start to include in your diet. Of course, if you are allergic to nuts, try seeds, or go for oils such as avocado or olive oil instead. Each of the foods included in this list support skin health either because of the key nutrients they contain or as a result of their impact on gut health. The recipes below include a variety of these foods and more, but do try to include some of these each day.

1 Avocadoes
2 Beans and lentils
3 Berries

4 Dark-green leafy vegetables
5 Fermented foods, such as kefir (see list on page 102)
6 Salmon
7 Tofu
8 Tomatoes
9 Turmeric
10 Walnuts and cashew nuts

The SkinFood storecupboard

Keeping the ingredients you need close to hand makes it so much easier to put a nourishing meal or snack together at a moment's notice. Below I have listed some staples that I recommend including in your shopping list and keeping stocked at home. Most should be readily available in a supermarket. Where I have included ingredients that are slightly less common, I have tried to add them to several recipes so that you aren't left with forgotten spices or herbs that you use only once. As a home cook (and I am certainly not a chef!) my aim is to make the SkinFood approach as accessible as possible, so it really has to be practical.

Greens

- Go for fresh or frozen fruit and vegetables.
- Supermarkets are fine, but think about farmers' markets or fresh fruit and veg boxes for a change, if you can.
- Look for a rainbow of colours in your shopping basket.
- Frozen berries are an excellent staple to keep on standby.
- Buy seasonal fruit and vegetables where possible, as this helps to maximise the nutrient content while

keeping costs down. An alternative is to stock up on frozen vegetables such as cauliflower, broccoli and spinach, which will retain their nutrients for longer than fresh options.

Lean proteins

- Tofu: look for firm/extra-firm fresh tofu packed in liquid.
- Tinned beans of any variety (such as chickpeas, green lentils): I tend to buy these in bulk online. You can get some of these in jars too, which are more expensive but delicious.
- Salmon: sustainable wild salmon is preferable.
- White fish: fresh or frozen, but again please do look for sustainable options where possible.
- Eggs, chicken and turkey: try to shop for organic or free-range sources if you can.
- Plain Greek yoghurt, ricotta or skyr (a Nordic strained yoghurt rich in protein).
- Quinoa, nuts and seeds also contain protein.

Oils and healthy fats

- Extra virgin olive oil is my go-to, but I also love avocado oil.
- Occasionally I use coconut oil in recipes (this should be virgin and cold pressed where possible).
- Cooking sprays (coconut or olive oil) are great for baking.
- Nuts can be purchased more economically in bulk

quantities online (1kg bags) and then stored in airtight containers.

- Seeds including ground flaxseeds, pumpkin seeds and sunflower seeds are a staple in many recipes.

Whole grains

- Sourdough or wholegrain seeded breads are preferable. Buckwheat, millet and other gluten-free breads are also rich in fibre.
- Wholegrain wraps and pitta bread.
- Brown rice, quinoa, whole-wheat bulgur and whole-wheat couscous (although the latter is not technically a whole grain; it is a lower glycaemic fibre-rich carbohydrate).
- Pouches of pre-cooked grains are helpful when you are pressed for time.
- When choosing pasta, look for wholegrain or experiment with pasta made from lentils, chickpeas or quinoa.
- Soba noodles are made from buckwheat flour – check to make sure that they are 100 per cent buckwheat if you are aiming for gluten-free.
- Oats: look for rolled oats (porridge oats), which are less processed.
- Flours for baking: whole-wheat flour, chickpea flour, buckwheat flour or, if you want gluten-free, your preferred choice.

Dairy and non-dairy

- Feta and halloumi cheese
- Live yoghurt
- Non-dairy cheese
- Non-dairy yoghurts (look for live yoghurt and yoghurt fortified with calcium and vitamins where possible).
- Parmesan cheese (which also contains probiotics; others listed below).

Probiotic and fermented foods

- Kefir
- Kimchi
- Miso (white) – a type of fermented soya bean paste
- Sauerkraut

(and see below)

Drinks

- Water: try infusing with lemon, lime, cucumber or mint to keep it interesting
- Chai tea
- Green tea or matcha
- Kombucha – a fermented tea rich in probiotics
- Herbal teas

Storecupboard staples

- Apricots (dried)

- Cinnamon (ground)
- Dates
- Harissa paste
- Honey
- Maple syrup
- Oatcakes
- Olives
- Turmeric (ground)
- Soy sauce (or tamari if you prefer gluten-free)

Breakfasts

Weekday breakfasts have to be quick and simple in our house, so my cacao goji granola and creamy oats are staples. But on weekends, or when there is more time, I love to whip up soft fluffy pancakes, crispy savoury frittatas or classic avocado and eggs on toast.

It's easy to skip breakfast if you're in rush, but taking the time to start your day with something nutritious allows you to feel energised. And what is nourishing food if not a little self-care?

If you are practising intermittent fasting and your breakfast is later in the day, many of these recipes are easily transportable or would work as brunch too.

BeautyFood Granola with Cacao and Goji

Making your own granola might seem daunting, but I assure you it will be love at first bite and well worth the effort. Once you have the ingredients to hand it actually takes much less time than you'd imagine to prepare. I make a batch at the weekend and store it in an airtight jar to keep it crisp, and then I can enjoy it over yoghurt with some fruit (GLOW-approved), or with ice-cold milk (which turns ever-so-satisfyingly chocolatey). It can also be saved for dessert and it is particularly delicious as a crunchy topping for ice cream, including the Avocado, Coconut and Lime Ice Cream on page 342.

As well as fibre-rich oats and good fats from nuts, this granola contains the antioxidant powerhouses cacao and goji berries, which have extraordinarily high levels of flavonoids; these fight inflammation and premature skin ageing. If you don't have access to these two ingredients, you can always use cocoa powder and dried cranberries or cherries instead.

Serves 10

275g rolled (porridge) oats

25g unsweetened desiccated coconut

150g raw nuts, chopped (I recommend walnuts and almonds). If omitting, increase oats by 50g instead

30g unsweetened cacao or cocoa powder

2 tbsp chia seeds

½ tsp sea salt

100ml maple syrup or honey

60ml coconut oil or olive oil

4 tbsp goji berries (dried cranberries or dried cherries also work well)

Preheat the oven to 200°C (180°C fan oven) Gas 6. Put the oats, coconut, nuts, cacao, chia seeds and salt into a food processor and pulse two or three times to combine. Transfer to a bowl. (Alternatively, if you don't have a food processor, you can mix the ingredients in a large bowl and combine using a wooden spoon, but the texture will be slightly crunchier.)

Warm the maple syrup with the oil in a small saucepan over

a medium-low heat to combine. Pour the mixture into the dry ingredients and stir well to ensure that everything is combined.

Spread the granola mix onto a large baking tray (you may need more than one) to make a thin, even layer, no more than 2cm thick. Cook in the oven for 10 minutes, then gently stir the granola to ensure it cooks evenly. Cook for a further 10 minutes. Allow the granola to fully cool before adding your dried berries. Store in an airtight container. It should keep for 1 week, but in our house it never lasts that long!

Glowing Green Juice

This is my absolute go-to green juice, especially when I'm feeling run down and needing an energy boost. If I've been on holiday and eaten nothing but croissants and fries for a week, I'll crave this juice and will have it with breakfast for a few days once I'm home. When I've been drinking it regularly, I genuinely feel that my skin looks better.

You don't need an expensive, state-of-the-art machine to make this – my juicer is small and compact, but it does the job. One thing to bear in mind, though, is that once you've made your green juice, it's best to drink it straightaway, as it will start to separate and change colour pretty quickly. If you're just making it for yourself, by all means cut the recipe quantities in half. And finally, you'll maximise the nutritional benefits of this juice by using the freshest ingredients you can find.

Serves 2–4
1 bunch of celery, roughly chopped
1 apple, cored and roughly chopped
1 pear, cored and roughly chopped

1 thumb-sized piece of fresh ginger, roughly chopped

2 big handfuls of spinach

1 cucumber, roughly chopped

juice of 1 lemon

Start by juicing your celery, apple, pear and ginger, before adding the spinach and finally the cucumber. The reason why the order is so specific is because the cucumber helps to 'flush' the spinach through the juicer so that there's as little wastage as possible.

Pour your juice into a jug and squeeze the juice of your lemon into it, then mix well.

If you aren't going to drink your juice immediately, make sure to chill it in an airtight bottle. Shake well before drinking.

Ricotta Toast – Three Ways

If you're someone who only ever has time for a slice of toast and jam in the morning, why not try substituting ricotta for the jam? Cool, creamy ricotta is deliciously protein-rich and forms the perfect basis of a deliciously simple breakfast. Below I've offered three different ways that you can enjoy this quick and easy meal, but feel free to experiment and come up with your own toppings – although make sure that you're including a variety of colours, textures and flavours. And if you are dairy-free, you can try a non-dairy cream cheese as an alternative to ricotta.

Serves 1

Topping 1

2 tbsp ricotta (mix in 1 tsp goat's cheese, if you like)

2 slices of wholegrain or seeded bread

a handful of cherry tomatoes, sliced

olive oil, to drizzle

a few basil leaves, torn

salt and ground black pepper

Spread a thick blanket of ricotta on your toast. Top with sliced cherry tomatoes, a drizzle of olive oil, a few torn basil leaves, and salt and pepper to taste.

Topping 2

2 tbsp ricotta

1 tsp honey

2 slices of wholegrain or seeded bread

1 nectarine, pitted and sliced

1 tbsp flaked almonds

Mix together the ricotta and honey, then spread it over your toast. Top with nectarine and a scattering of almonds.

Variation

This is particularly good with nectarines that have been lightly browned in a pan, if you have the time.

Topping 3

2 tbsp ricotta

1 tsp chives, chopped

1 tsp dill leaves, chopped

2 slices of wholegrain or seeded bread

1 generous slice smoked salmon

1 tsp lemon juice

1 radish (optional), sliced

salt and ground black pepper

This is a lighter take on the deli favourite, smoked salmon and cream cheese. Mix the ricotta with the chopped herbs and season to taste with salt and pepper. Spread the herby ricotta on your toast and top with the smoked salmon and a squeeze of lemon juice to finish. If you are a radish fan, add a thin layer of sliced radish to give your toast extra dimension and colour.

Masala Scrambled Eggs

This breakfast will transport you to the bustling heart of Mumbai in an instant. A cup of warming chai is the perfect accompaniment. Eggs are protein- and vitamin-rich, and the warming spices in both the eggs and chai have numerous anti-inflammatory benefits.

Serves 2

1 tsp olive oil

2 spring onions, finely sliced

1 ripe tomato, roughly chopped

1 green chilli, deseeded and sliced

1 tbsp chopped coriander leaves

½ tsp ground cumin

½ tsp ground coriander

a pinch of ground turmeric

4 large eggs, beaten

toasted pitta, whole-wheat wrap or chapatti (optional), to serve

Heat the oil in a non-stick pan over a medium heat, then cook the spring onions for 2–3 minutes. Add the tomato, chilli, fresh coriander and spices, and stir well, mashing the tomato as you go. After about 3–4 minutes the mixture should be fragrant and soft. Reduce the heat to medium-low and stir in the beaten eggs, folding them gently until they are cooked to your liking.

You can either enjoy your eggs on their own, or create a more substantial breakfast by enveloping them in a toasted wholegrain pitta, wrap or chapatti.

BeauTea Chai

This warming spiced tea is the lifeblood of India and Sri Lanka. It is drunk by everyone, regardless of their social status, throughout the day. Its roots lie in Ayurveda, and the original recipe can be traced back over 5,000 years.

I may be biased, but in my opinion the most beautiful tea is Ceylon, and much of it is grown in the lush hillsides surrounding Nuwara Eliya (close to where I was born). This leaf tea is particularly high in catechins and theaflavins, which have remarkable anti-inflammatory and antioxidant properties. Combined with the most fragrant spices, it serves as an instant pick-me-up.

Serves 2

5 cardamom pods

3 cloves

4 peppercorns

½ cinnamon stick

3 thin slices of peeled fresh ginger

1 tbsp Ceylon leaf tea or a teabag

250ml milk of choice

sweetener of choice (such as honey, maple syrup, sugar, coconut sugar)

Pour 250ml water into a saucepan and place over a low heat. Gently crush the cardamom pods, cloves and peppercorns using a pestle and mortar before adding them to your saucepan along with the cinnamon stick and sliced ginger.

Once the water is gently simmering, put a lid on your saucepan and let it simmer for 10 minutes to make the chai base.

Turn off the heat and add your tea leaves to the base. Leave to infuse for 5 minutes, then add your milk of choice and bring the tea back to a simmer. Finally, sweeten to taste before straining and pouring the tea into a teacup.

Feta Frittata with Spring Vegetables

This gorgeously sunny frittata is delicious hot or cold. Leftovers make the perfect lunch with a salad or tomato salsa. I've gone for asparagus and peas in mine, but you can be flexible with your choice of vegetables – courgettes and peppers also work very well. This meal is GLOW on a plate.

Serves 4
1 small bunch of asparagus
1 tbsp olive oil
1 small shallot, finely sliced
8 eggs, beaten
100g feta cheese, crumbled
100g frozen peas, defrosted
2 tbsp chopped fresh herbs, such as chives and basil
a pinch of dried chilli flakes
salt and ground black pepper
wholegrain bread and a dressed tomato salad (optional), to serve

Remove the woody asparagus ends by bending them to locate their tender snapping point. Slice the asparagus diagonally but keep the tips intact.

Heat the oil in a 20cm non-stick frying pan over a medium heat.

Add the shallot and cook for 5 minutes until softened. Add the sliced asparagus. The asparagus should stay bright green, so cook it for no longer than 5 minutes.

Season the beaten eggs with salt and pepper, add the feta, peas, herbs and chilli and mix well.

Pour the egg mixture into your frying pan and mix together the ingredients. Continue to cook over a medium heat for 10 minutes. Meanwhile preheat the grill.

Put the pan under the hot grill and cook for 5–10 minutes until puffed and golden.

Allow your frittata to cool before slicing, and enjoy. To create a heartier meal, you can serve with wholegrain bread and a tomato salad that's simply dressed with a little red wine vinegar and olive oil.

Five-Minute Banana Oat Pancakes

These are so quick to make that even a weekday breakfast can feel like a weekend brunch! Oats and bananas provide slow-releasing energy and help to keep blood sugar levels stable, so they are a great sweet breakfast option.

Serves 2–4
2 ripe bananas
2 eggs
120ml milk of your choice
1 tsp vanilla extract
½ tsp ground cinnamon
120g rolled (porridge) oats
2 tsp baking powder

a pinch of salt

coconut, avocado or olive oil, for frying

yoghurt, fresh berries, sliced almonds and a drizzle of
honey, maple or date syrup (optional), to serve

Put all the ingredients, except the oil, into a blender or food
processor and blend on high until you have a completely smooth
mixture. Leave to stand for 1 minute.

While your pancake mix is resting, heat a little oil in a non-stick frying
pan over a medium heat. Add 1 tbsp of mix per pancake to the pan
and allow them to puff up for 2–4 minutes until nice and golden, then
flip them over and cook for another 2–4 minutes until golden.

These pancakes are delicious eaten on their own, but I also love
to serve them with yoghurt, fresh berries, almonds and a drizzle of
honey, maple or date syrup.

Beauty Bowl: Creamy Porridge with Pistachio and Cherries

This deliciously creamy porridge is everything you want in
a breakfast: it's quick, easy and versatile. Oats are fibre-rich
whole grains, loved by our gut bacteria. They also release energy
slowly, which allows you to stay feeling full.

When it comes to toppings, the choices are endless. My personal go-to is a combination of fruit and nuts/seeds to make
this a balanced GLOW bowl. With their dark, juicy sweetness
cherries are chock-full of antioxidant anthocyanins, while pistachio nuts add crunch, protein and healthy fats. You could make
double or triple the quantity of cherry compote to enjoy throughout the week – it's gorgeous over yoghurt or pancakes too.

I use traditional rolled (porridge) oats, as these are less processed, but they can take a little longer to prepare. This is a

recipe from my mother, who is fastidious about her daily bowl of oats, and it involves soaking to ensure that your porridge has a creamy finish.

Serves 1
40g rolled (porridge) oats
a handful of frozen cherries
juice of ½ orange
½ tsp honey, plus extra to serve (optional)
a pinch of salt
100ml milk of your choice
2–3 tsp pistachio nuts, to taste, chopped

Pour 175ml water into a small saucepan over a high heat and bring to the boil. Take the pan off the heat, then add your oats and stir. Leave for 10 minutes.

Meanwhile, put the frozen cherries in a separate saucepan over a low heat, squashing them with a fork as they cook. Add the honey and orange juice and cook for 10 minutes or until gently softened, to create a cherry compote.

Add the salt and milk to the oats and bring to the boil over a medium heat, stirring regularly, for about 5 minutes. You can adjust the consistency of the porridge to suit your taste by adding a little more milk.

Pour the porridge into a bowl, top with the cherry compote and sprinkle over the chopped nuts.

Variations
If you want to keep your porridge interesting, here are some other great topping combinations:

- Fresh berries and mixed seeds
- Mango and desiccated coconut (particularly good with porridge made with coconut milk)
- Sliced figs and granola
- Poached apple, cinnamon and pecan nuts
- Fresh apricots, vanilla and ground flaxseeds

Sweetcorn Fritters with Avocado Smash

These crispy spicy fritters are wonderful when you have a little more time on your hands, and they are great with a poached egg too. Sweetcorn is full of fibre and contains two key nutrients, lutein and zeaxanthin, which boost skin health by protecting against UV damage. Creamy-rich avocado adds more skin-loving healthy fats.

Serves 4

2 tablespoons whole-wheat/brown flour (or any gluten-free flour)
½ tsp baking powder
2 eggs
2 tbsp milk
2 spring onions, finely sliced
250g sweetcorn (I use defrosted frozen corn)
½ red chilli, deseeded and finely chopped
a handful of coriander leaves, chopped
1 avocado
juice of 1 lime, plus 1 lime cut into quarters
1 tbsp olive oil
salt and ground black pepper
chilli sauce and yoghurt (optional), to serve

Place the flour and baking powder in a large mixing bowl. In another bowl gently whisk the eggs together with the milk before combining with the flour mixture.

Add the spring onions, sweetcorn, chilli and coriander, and generously season with salt and pepper. Leave the batter to stand for 5 minutes.

In the meantime, in a medium-sized bowl, smash the avocado flesh with a fork and season with salt, pepper and lime juice.

Once the batter is ready, heat the oil in a large frying pan over a medium heat. Add a heaped tablespoon of the batter for each fritter, patting down with the spoon to make rounds. Pan-fry gently until golden on both sides – this takes about 2 minutes per side. This mixture makes approximately eight fritters.

Finish by serving the fritters with your avocado smash and a lime quarter on each portion. You can also add some chilli sauce and yoghurt on the side, if you like.

Glow Gorgeous Cherry Cashew Smoothie

I devised this recipe to help support healthy skin and hair. Our hair is very sensitive to nutrition, and increased hair shedding can be caused by low iron, B12, protein and even low-calorie diets or rapid weight loss. A balanced diet is essential to promoting skin and hair health.

Spinach is one of the richest plant sources of iron, one of the most important minerals for hair health, while cherries provide vitamin C, which helps to improve iron absorption. Nut butters are full of zinc, selenium, protein and healthy fats. I've added collagen powder to this smoothie, as there is early evidence it may improve skin smoothness and hydration, but it isn't a must by any means.

Serves 1

250ml milk of choice

40g baby leaf spinach

1 tsp nut butter

½ ripe banana

a large handful of frozen cherries

1 date

1–2 tbsp collagen powder (optional)

This is a simple one: add all the ingredients to a blender and blend until smooth. Enjoy!

Golden Sunshine Smoothie

By now you probably know that I adore turmeric, not only for its deeply golden warmth but also for its incredible nutritional profile. This all-round wonder spice has been prized for centuries for its extraordinary anti-inflammatory properties. As children, we were encouraged to drink turmeric milk to fight off colds, and pastes of turmeric were applied to cuts and grazes. Science has slowly caught up, and more than 1,000 research papers have studied this truly remarkable spice.

A little black pepper helps to boost the absorption of curcumin, the active anti-inflammatory ingredient in turmeric, and I would also try adding a few dried rose petals to this smoothie to make it as beautiful as it is delicious.

Serves 1

140g frozen mango

250ml milk of choice (I recommend coconut for this recipe)

2 tbsp yoghurt/kefir of choice

a pinch of ground black pepper

¼ tsp ground turmeric

2–3 drops of rosewater, to taste

a few dried rose petals (optional)

Blend together the ingredients, except the dried rose petals (if using), in a blender. Pour into a glass and top with dried rose petals and enjoy ice cold.

Yoghurt with Plum and Vanilla Compote

Live yoghurt is full of probiotic bacteria that are essential for gut health. You can choose whichever yoghurt you prefer for this recipe, but I like to use varieties such as Greek or skyr, as they contain more protein, which helps us to feel sated and supports strong skin, hair and nails.

The compote is best made with ripe, sweet plums so that you don't need to add too much extra sugar, and a squeeze of orange adds a bright note. If you're not a yoghurt person, this compote is also lovely over porridge.

Serves 2

250g ripe sweet plums (about 5 or 6), halved and pitted

juice of ½ orange

1 tsp vanilla extract

½ tsp ground cinnamon

1 tsp honey or sweetener of choice

300g yoghurt of choice

1 tbsp roasted hazelnuts, chopped

Cut the plums in half again so that you have quarter segments.

Put the segments in a saucepan with 2 tbsp water and heat over a medium-low heat for 10–15 minutes to allow the plums to gently soften.

Add the orange juice, vanilla, cinnamon and sweetener to the saucepan and continue to heat on medium for a further 5 minutes.

Gently mash some of the plums with a spoon to ensure a soft compote. Leave to cool slightly before serving over cool yoghurt and top with hazelnuts.

Lunches

You might be in the habit of grabbing a quick sandwich for lunch, but I find that all too often this leads to a slump in energy and sugar cravings by 4pm. In this section you'll find warming soups, hearty salads and flavour-packed sandwiches too, all designed with GLOW in mind, to keep you feeling satisfied and your blood sugar stabilised.

Make sure to take the time to sit and eat your lunch properly if you can, rather than snatching quick bites at your desk. Eating slowly and chewing properly helps to aid digestion and prevents bloating and discomfort after meals.

Creamy Chestnut Mushroom and Porcini Soup

The humble mushroom really is quite incredible. With over 400 varieties, mushrooms have been central to traditional Chinese medicine for thousands of years. Research into these seemingly unassuming fungi has shown their amazing ability to protect brain health, and their impact on stemming cancer-cell growth is also being investigated.

In this recipe, I've gone for chestnut and porcini mushrooms, because they are readily available, but please do feel free to experiment with different varieties that you come across. You won't taste the cannellini beans in this soup, but they add a rich, creamy texture as well as protein.

Serves 4

500g chestnut mushrooms

15g dried porcini mushrooms

700ml vegetable stock

1 tbsp nutritional yeast

2 tbsp olive oil

1 leek, chopped

2 garlic cloves, chopped

4 thyme sprigs

400g tin cannellini beans, drained and rinsed

salt and ground black pepper

dried chilli flakes, pumpkin seeds and parsley,
with bread of choice, to serve

Discard the stalks from the chestnut mushrooms and slice the caps. Put the dried porcini in a measuring jug and add 200ml of boiling water and nutritional yeast, stir well.

Heat the olive oil in a heavy-based saucepan over a medium heat. Add the chopped leek and allow it to soften for 5 minutes, then add the garlic and stir. Next add the chestnut mushrooms and thyme, and stir to ensure that everything is well combined. Season well with salt and pepper.

Put the lid on the pan and let the mushrooms soften over a medium-low heat for 15 minutes. Then add the cannellini beans and the vegetable stock and porcini mix. Leave to simmer gently for a further 15 minutes.

Season to taste and blend using a high-speed or hand-held blender. I top this with chilli flakes, pumpkin seeds and parsley, and scoop it up with warm sourdough bread.

Tuscan White Bean Soup

This hearty, comforting soup uses an array of vegetables, so I often make it, or a version of it, when I'm trying to clear out the fridge. It is also economical to make and stores well, tasting even better the next day. It may seem rather simple, but it's a daily staple in many Mediterranean countries – and it's dishes like this that are thought to contribute to living a long and healthy life.

To create extra depth of flavour, I add nutritional yeast, which also boosts levels of B vitamins that are key for skin and hair health. When serving, I love topping with a generous heap of Parmesan, which gives the soup a lovely added richness and supports gut health. If you want to change things up, you can also try finishing with the Walnut Pesto on page 326 and this adds an extra hit of skin-friendly good fats.

Serves 4 (generously)

2 tbsp olive oil, plus extra for drizzling

1 onion, chopped

2 carrots, chopped

2 celery sticks, chopped

4 garlic cloves, chopped

2 bay leaves

leaves from 4 thyme sprigs

2 × 400g tins cannellini beans, drained and rinsed

2 tbsp tomato purée

1 tsp dried chilli flakes

800ml vegetable stock

1 tbsp nutritional yeast

100g kale, spinach or cavolo nero, shredded

salt and ground black pepper

grated Parmesan or vegan cheese, bread of
choice, Walnut Pesto (page 326), to serve

Heat the oil in a large heavy-based pan over a medium heat. Add
the onion and cook for 5 minutes or until softened and translucent.

Add the carrots, celery and garlic. Mix well and cook for a further
10 minutes.

Add the bay leaves, thyme, cannellini beans, tomato purée and chilli
flakes, and season with salt and pepper to taste. Mix well.

Stir in the stock and nutritional yeast, then bring to the boil. Reduce
the heat and leave to simmer, covered, over a medium-low heat for
20 minutes to let the flavours meld.

Finally, add your chosen greens and let these cook for a further
5 minutes. This soup is chunky, and that's just how I like it, but if
you prefer a smoother soup, take the bay leaves out and blend
before serving.

Serve in large bowls with a drizzle of olive oil, a generous grating of
Parmesan, some warm bread and a dollop of walnut pesto.

Radiant Roasted Tomato Soup with Crunchy Croutons

Tomatoes are one of my top-ten skin foods, and it makes perfect
sense given their many health benefits. They are nature's richest
source of lycopene, an incredibly potent antioxidant carotenoid
that has been shown to protect the skin against ageing and UV
damage when cooked.

This recipe will allow you to make the most of your tomatoes, as the roasting process brings out their natural sweet flavour, even if they aren't beautifully ripe to begin with. It's also refreshingly simple, so you can whip up a hearty lunch in no time at all!

Serves 2

400g tomatoes (I like to use a mix of varieties, such as cherry and plum), chopped into large chunks if large

3 garlic cloves, unpeeled

½ red onion, sliced

1 tbsp olive oil

250ml vegetable stock

salt and ground black pepper

25g feta, crumbled

4 basil leaves, torn, to garnish

For the croutons:

2 slices of wholegrain bread (it works best slightly stale), cut into chunks

1 tbsp olive oil

salt and ground black pepper

Preheat the oven to 200°C (180°C fan oven) Gas 6 and line a baking tray. Put the tomatoes on the prepared baking tray and add the garlic and sliced red onion. Season with salt and pepper, and drizzle with the olive oil. Roast for 20–30 minutes until soft.

To make the croutons, coat the bread chunks in the oil and season with salt and pepper to taste. Put on a baking tray and bake for 7–10 minutes until crisp, turning once half-way through.

Squeeze the cloves of roasted garlic out of their skins and add to a blender or food processor along with the tomatoes and onion. Add the vegetable stock and crumbled feta. Blend until smooth. Pour into a saucepan and gently reheat.

Ladle into bowls and garnish with torn basil leaves. Serve with the crunchy croutons.

Eat to GLOW Mix-and-Match Grain Bowl

This salad is a lifesaver when you're in a rush, as all it takes is a little prep on a Sunday. It saves you time, money and packs a nutrient-dense hit – plus it tastes delicious, and I find it so much more satisfying than a shop-bought salad.

To put it together all you have to do is pick ingredients from each of the GLOW categories. I've listed my favourite skin-loving ingredients below, which I highly recommend you try, but it can be as simple as using whatever you have in the fridge. Some sauerkraut or kimchi on the side makes a gut-boosting addition.

Add a selection from each of the following categories:

Greens Tomatoes, cucumber, beetroot, celery, radish, carrot, leftover roasted veg, olives
Lean protein Halloumi, feta, tofu, chickpeas, lentils, leftover salmon, chicken or tuna
Oils and healthy fats Avocados, nuts, seeds, olive oil, avocado oil
Whole grain The recipe is for bulgur wheat, but you can also use quinoa, whole-wheat couscous, brown rice, whole-wheat pasta

Serves 4
200g uncooked bulgur wheat
125g (½ block) halloumi cheese, diced

2 tbsp olive oil, plus a little extra for frying

½ large cucumber, deseeded and chopped into chunks

125g cherry tomatoes

a large handful of parsley leaves, chopped

½ red onion, chopped

400g tin chickpeas, drained and rinsed

50g shelled unsalted pistachio nuts

juice of 1 lemon

salt and ground black pepper

Cook the bulgur wheat according to packet instructions and then fluff up the grains with a fork. Allow to cool.

Lightly brown the halloumi in a frying pan with a little oil over a medium heat. Set aside to cool.

In a large salad bowl combine the cooked bulgur, halloumi, salad vegetables, parsley, onion, chickpeas and nuts, and mix well. Dress with the lemon juice and the 2 tbsp oil, and season to taste with salt and pepper. If you like your food extra lemony, as I do, feel free to add more lemon juice.

Store in the fridge in an airtight container to enjoy for lunch all week. It's also a great side-salad alongside simply cooked chicken or fish.

Seared Salmon with a Crunchy Lentil Salad

It will come as no surprise that salmon is one of my favourite skin foods. It is rich in healthy fats and is a source of complete protein, which makes it essential for the repair and maintenance of the skin, hair and nails. It is also one of the richest sources of astaxanthin, which gives it its pink colour. You may not have

heard of astaxanthin, but it is thought that its powerful antioxi
dants play a role in helping freshwater salmon leap upstream
against the currents. Fortunately, as humans we aren't quite so
up against it, but by eating salmon twice a week, we can reap the
benefits for our skin and hair. If you can, look for sustainably
caught wild salmon, which also happens to have higher levels of
omega-3 and astaxanthin than farmed varieties.

Serves 2

400g tin green lentils, drained and rinsed (or 100g
dried green/Puy lentils, cooked for 30 minutes)

2 carrots, diced

2 celery sticks, diced

1 red pepper, deseeded and diced

¼ red onion, diced

2 tbsp mint leaves, chopped

2 tbsp olive oil, plus extra for frying

juice of ½ lemon, plus extra to serve

1 tsp honey

1 tsp mustard

2 salmon fillets

salt and ground black pepper

Put the lentils in a large salad bowl and add the carrots, celery, red
pepper, red onion and chopped mint.

Make the salad dressing by combining the 2 tbsp of oil with the
lemon juice, honey and mustard. Add salt and pepper to taste.
Drizzle the dressing over your salad ingredients and mix well to
combine. Set aside while you prepare the salmon.

Pat the salmon fillets dry with kitchen paper and season with salt
and pepper.

Heat a little olive oil in a heavy-based frying pan over a medium-high heat. Once the oil is hot, put the salmon skin-side down in the pan and cook for 4–5 minutes until crisp, before turning it over and cooking for a further 3–4 minutes until cooked through and the flesh flakes easily.

Transfer to a plate. Add a generous serving of the lentil salad and an extra squeeze of lemon. You may well have some lentil salad left over for lunch the next day too!

Roasted Beetroot and Butternut Salad with Feta and Hazelnuts

This salad is a million miles away from a Tupperware of limp lettuce leaves. Rich, vibrant and delicious, this salad will make you feel enlivened just by looking at it. 'Eat the rainbow' might sound a little clichéd, but by eating a range of colourful foods, such as the orange squash and the deeply purple beetroot in this recipe, you're supplying your body with a variety of different nutrients, each with its own benefits. Be generous with the hazelnuts as they add crunch and good fats, but if you're not a huge fan of how they taste you can substitute some lightly toasted pumpkin seeds for them instead.

Serves 2–3

2 tbsp olive oil

1 tbsp honey

350g butternut squash, diced

1 red onion, cut into thin wedges

2 garlic cloves, unpeeled

3 raw beetroot, peeled and cut into large chunks

40g raw hazelnuts

80g rocket leaves
75g feta or vegan cheese, crumbled
salt and ground black pepper

For the dressing:
1 tbsp balsamic vinegar
1 tsp honey
2 tbsp olive oil

Preheat the oven to 220°C (200°C fan oven) Gas 7. Mix the olive oil and honey in a large bowl, then add the squash, red onion, garlic cloves and beetroot. Season with salt and black pepper to taste and toss the vegetables to ensure that they are well coated and glistening.

Spread your vegetables evenly over a large baking tray and pop in the oven for 30–40 minutes until golden and roasted.

Put the hazelnuts on a separate tray and toast in the oven for 4–5 minutes maximum – if left for longer they will burn and taste bitter.

In a small bowl, squeeze the roasted garlic cloves out of their skin and mash with a fork until smooth. Add the dressing ingredients and mix until well combined. Season with salt and pepper.

To assemble the salad, start with a base layer of rocket leaves on a large plate, followed by the roasted vegetables and the crumbled feta, and finish with the hazelnuts and a generous drizzle of the balsamic dressing.

Three make-ahead salads

I love to prepare a protein-based salad at the weekend, and one that keeps well in the fridge all week. It can be added to a simple leaf salad, some quickly boiled new potatoes or atop a slice of toasted bread. I've included my three favourite versions over the following pages, each balanced with protein, good fats and crunchy vegetables.

Turmeric Roasted Chicken Salad

This golden chicken salad is a twist on the classic coronation chicken. I've added extra oomph with smoky turmeric-baked chicken and a tangy yoghurt dressing.

Serves 2–4

2 chicken breasts

2 tbsp live yoghurt

1 tbsp avocado mayonnaise or regular mayonnaise

1 tbsp mango chutney

1 tsp maple syrup

2 celery sticks, diced

a handful of red seedless grapes, halved

1 spring onion, finely sliced

2 tbsp flaked almonds

For the marinade:

1 tbsp olive oil

1 tsp ground turmeric

1 tsp ginger paste or 1cm fresh ginger, peeled and grated

1 tsp garlic paste or 1 garlic clove, crushed

salt and ground black pepper

Mix together the marinade ingredients in a bowl and use to massage the chicken breasts to coat them generously. Leave to stand for 30 minutes.

Preheat the oven to 200°C (180°C fan oven) Gas 6. Put the chicken on a baking tray and cook for 30 minutes or until tender and cooked through. Allow the chicken to cool completely.

While the chicken is cooking, create the salad dressing by mixing together the yoghurt, mayonnaise, mango chutney and maple syrup until smooth.

Shred the chicken breast. Put the celery and grapes in a large bowl and add the shredded chicken, spring onion and flaked almonds. Stir in the dressing and toss together using salad tongs to ensure that everything is well combined. Finish by seasoning with salt and pepper to taste.

Salmon Salad with Capers, Dill and Lemon

This recipe was inspired by a delicious Scandinavian-style sandwich I ate recently at Pret a Manger: layers of smoked salmon, dill and a tangy mustard mayo ensconced in a chewy rye bun. I wanted to make something that was altogether more in keeping with the principles of the SkinFood approach, with plenty of skin-friendly salmon and added celery for crunch. I really hope you enjoy it!

This salad works really well piled high on toasted rye, but by all means feel free to experiment and come up with your own combinations. It keeps well in the fridge for up to 4 days.

Serves 2
2 salmon fillets about 120g each, or 210g tin wild sustainable salmon
a little olive oil
2 tbsp yoghurt
1 tsp mayonnaise
½ tsp English mustard
juice of ½ lemon

¼ red onion, finely chopped

2 celery sticks, diced

1 tbsp capers, chopped

2 tbsp dill fronds, finely chopped

salt and black pepper

If you are using fresh salmon fillets, preheat the oven to 200°C (180°C fan oven) Gas 6. Rub the fillets with olive oil, season with salt and pepper and then cook in the oven for 20 minutes until cooked through and the flesh flakes easily. Allow the salmon to cool before breaking it up into large flakes using a fork. If you have opted for tinned salmon (which is an excellent storecupboard staple), you are ready to move straight on to the next step.

Mix together the yoghurt, mayonnaise, mustard and lemon juice until well combined. Add the chopped onion, celery, capers and dill. Gently fold through the salmon to prevent the flakes from completely disintegrating. Season with salt and pepper to your liking.

Either enjoy immediately or store in an airtight container in the fridge for up to 4 days.

Chickpea 'Tuna' Salad Sandwich

This is quite possibly my favourite vegan sandwich filling. I stumbled upon it quite accidentally, as one so often does, after some late-night Instagram scrolling. I am always looking for ways to include more beans and pulses in my diet, and this is a delicious way to do this.

I am not vegan but I do enjoy vegan food immensely. My mother is vegetarian, so as a child I grew up enjoying vegan food before it became as mainstream as it is now.

This filling is delicious, tangy and moreish – and every time I make it, I have to stop myself from scraping the bowl. I love it spread on a toasted wholegrain seeded bagel with a few slices of tomato, red onion for a cool crunch and a little sliced avocado.

Serves 2

400g tin chickpeas, drained and rinsed
1 celery stick, finely chopped
¼ red onion, finely chopped
2 tsp capers, chopped
¼ tsp garlic paste or ¼ garlic clove, crushed
1 tbsp vegan mayonnaise (or yoghurt if preferred)
juice of ½ lemon
a splash of Tabasco sauce
salt and ground black pepper

To serve:
2 whole-wheat seeded bagels
½ red onion, sliced
1 tomato, sliced
½ avocado, sliced

Put the chickpeas in a large mixing bowl and gently break them up using a fork. Make sure not to overdo it, as you don't want to end up with a chickpea paste! Add the remaining ingredients and season to taste with salt and pepper. Mix well so that the ingredients are properly combined.

Pile high onto the toasted bagels, layer with thin slices of red onion, tomato and avocado. Eat immediately.

Light and Bright Rainbow Noodle Salad with Crispy Tofu

Food is just as much about texture as it is flavour. After perfecting this recipe over numerous iterations, I've finally managed to get the tofu as crispy as it can be. I love to combine my tofu with this gorgeously bright noodle salad, but it works just as well as the protein component of a mix-and-match GLOW bowl, or as a side to a simple meal of rice and broccoli.

Tofu is a complete source of protein, meaning that it has all the amino acids required by the body for repair and regeneration. Many of us don't get enough protein in our diet, and as our skin, hair and nails are fundamentally built of protein, it's a key requirement. Tofu and other soya-based foods contain soy isoflavones, a type of phyto-oestrogen that fights skin ageing; in fact, you'll find soy isoflavones as a skincare ingredient in many anti-ageing products.

For the noodle salad, look for whole-wheat, brown rice or buckwheat soba noodles to increase fibre and B-vitamin content. There is a bit more chopping required in this recipe than in others, but I assure you it's worth it for this gorgeously colourful salad. This recipe very generously serves two, but leftovers are never a bad thing in my book. It's also easily scalable and it is always a hit when feeding a crowd.

Serves 2–4

1 block extra-firm tofu (about 300g), drained

1 tbsp extra-virgin olive oil

1 tbsp soy sauce or tamari if you are gluten-free

1 tbsp cornflour

a handful of cashew nuts, chopped (optional), to serve

For the rainbow noodle salad:

150g soba noodles (or whole-wheat noodle of choice)

½ cucumber, deseeded and julienned

1 red pepper, deseeded and julienned

1 carrot, julienned

100g edamame beans (I use frozen, thawed)

¼ red cabbage, thinly sliced

4 spring onions, thinly sliced

a handful of coriander leaves, roughly chopped

½ red chilli, deseeded and finely chopped

salt

For the dressing:

juice of 1 lime

2cm piece of fresh ginger, peeled and grated

1 clove garlic, grated

1 tsp miso paste

1 tsp sesame oil (replace with olive oil if allergic)

1½ tbsp soy sauce

1 tbsp honey or maple syrup

Preheat the oven to 220°C (200°C fan oven) Gas 7. Cut the tofu into 2cm cubes and coat in the oil and soy sauce. Sprinkle over the cornflour and mix well until evenly coated. Place in the oven on a baking sheet for 20 minutes, tossing halfway through to ensure even crunchiness.

Cook the soba noodles in a saucepan of boiling water according to the pack instructions. Drain well and rinse under cold water, set aside and leave to cool.

Put the remaining salad ingredients in a large salad bowl and add the noodles.

Mix together the dressing ingredients then pour it over the salad. Top with the crispy tofu and the cashew nuts (if using).

Green Chickpea Pancakes with Mushrooms and Kimchi

These luminous green pancakes are a popular breakfast dish known as *besan chilla*. They are naturally vegan and made with chickpea flour, which is widely used in Indian and Sri Lankan cooking, where it's often referred to as gram flour. This is my version, stuffed with mushrooms and probiotic-rich kimchi, but sauerkraut is an equally microbe-enhancing alternative. This is a feast for both the taste buds and the gut microbes and, as you now know, gut health and skin health are closely intertwined.

Serves 2

100g chickpea flour

275ml water

a handful of spinach

a handful of green herbs (I like coriander)

a pinch of salt

1 tbsp olive, coconut or avocado oil, plus extra for frying

For the filling:

1 tbsp olive oil

1 garlic clove, crushed

250g mushrooms (I like chestnut), sliced

1 avocado, sliced

1 tbsp kimchi per pancake

salt and ground black pepper

Combine the chickpea flour, water, spinach, herbs, salt and oil in a blender until you have a relatively thin, smooth batter. Leave this to rest for 5 minutes.

Heat a little oil in a large frying pan over a medium-high heat and then coat the pan with a thin layer of batter. It should take only a minute for the batter to set and its surface to bubble. Flip the pancake and, once cooked through, slide it onto a plate. Repeat this process until you have finished your batter.

To make the filling, heat the olive oil in a saucepan over a medium-low heat and cook the garlic and mushrooms for 10 minutes or until softened. Season with salt and pepper to taste.

Fill the pancakes with the mushroom mixture, sliced avocado and 1 tbsp kimchi per pancake.

Main meals

At the end of a busy day, sitting down to a delicious meal is one of life's most simple pleasures. Although we're often pressed for time when it comes to preparing breakfast and lunch, dinner offers an opportunity to play and experiment a little more – it's when food can be at its most exciting and inventive.

Many of the following recipes can be easily stored in the freezer and reheated, so there's as little wastage as possible and you are always only minutes away from a tasty meal. I try to keep pouches of microwaveable grains in the cupboard to serve on the side along with a few slices of avocado for healthy fat and a spoonful of kimchi for probiotic-laden spice to create a 5-minute GLOW meal.

Soothing Sri Lankan Dhal with Kefir Raita

My mother has made the most delicious, quick-cook Sri-Lankan dhal (*parippu*) for decades. This is one of my favourite comfort meals: a hug in a bowl. There are recipes that involve soaking lentils for hours, but as a working mum herself, she found tricks to maximise flavour without losing authenticity. Red lentils are enriched with fibre, protein and minerals, and by now you'll know that I am fanatical about spices such as turmeric and cinnamon.

This simple dish can be served alone with rice or with turmeric roast chicken (page 311) or pan-fried prawns seasoned with a little salt and chilli powder. The kefir raita adds freshness and a welcome hit of probiotics, but you could also replace it with your preferred live yoghurt instead.

Serves 4

200g red lentils

1 tsp ginger paste or 1cm fresh ginger, peeled and grated

1 tsp ground turmeric

1 tsp ground cumin

½ tsp ground coriander

1–2 tsp red chilli powder (omit if you want a milder taste)

1 small green chilli, halved

3 garlic cloves, finely chopped

2 tsp salt

1 small red onion, chopped

1 small tomato, chopped

125ml full-fat coconut milk

brown rice or whole-wheat chapattis, to serve

For the kefir raita:

1 cucumber, chopped

350g kefir yoghurt or yoghurt of choice

1 tsp ground cumin

2 tbsp fresh mint or coriander leaves

salt and ground black pepper

For the tempered oil:

1 tbsp olive, avocado or coconut oil

1 tsp mustard seeds

½ tsp cumin seeds

50g cashew nuts

5 curry leaves (optional)

Rinse the lentils very well in water, draining and washing two to three times until the water runs clear. Put the lentils in a heavy-based saucepan and add 600ml water, the spices, garlic, ginger, salt, onion and tomato, and bring to the boil. Reduce the heat to a simmer, cover with a lid and cook for 10–15 minutes until the water evaporates. Add the coconut milk and stir well to combine over a medium heat.

While the lentils are cooking, you can prepare the raita by mixing together the ingredients in a small bowl.

To make the tempered oil, heat the oil in a small frying pan over a medium-high heat, then add the spices and cook, stirring, for 2–3 minutes until aromatic. Finally, add the cashews and curry leaves (if using) and lightly brown.

Pour the sizzling spice mix over the dhal and stir to combine. Serve with the raita, brown rice or whole-wheat chapattis.

Harissa-Spiced Turkey Burgers with Sweet Potato Wedges
and a Red Cabbage Slaw

These deliciously moist and flavoursome burgers are better than
any takeaway. Turkey meat is very lean but protein-rich, while
sweet potatoes contain B vitamins, iron and magnesium as well
as beta-carotene to create a nutrient-rich meal.

If you want to change this recipe, try making these burgers
into meatballs or koftas instead, and serve with warm pitta and
a generous amount of hummus.

Serves 4
400g minced turkey (either breast or thigh)
1 egg
2 tbsp harissa paste
3 garlic cloves, grated
1 tbsp olive oil

For the sweet potato wedges:
4 sweet potatoes, unpeeled and cut into wedges
2 tsp ground cumin
1 tbsp olive oil
salt and ground black pepper

For the red cabbage slaw:
¼ red cabbage, finely sliced
2 tbsp yoghurt
50g walnuts, chopped
50g dried cranberries
1 tbsp vinegar (I use apple cider vinegar)

Preheat the oven to 220°C (200°C fan oven) Gas 7. Coat the sweet potatoes in salt, pepper, the cumin and olive oil. Spread onto a baking sheet and bake for 30–40 minutes until crispy.

Put the minced turkey in a large bowl and add the egg, harissa paste and garlic. Mix well. Form into patties – you should have enough to create 4 larger ones or 8 mini ones. Leave in the fridge to set for 30 minutes.

In the meantime, mix together the slaw ingredients in a bowl and set aside.

Heat the 1 tbsp oil in a frying pan over a medium heat, add the turkey burgers and cook for 5–7 minutes on each side until cooked through. Serve with the sweet potato wedges and slaw on the side.

Lentil and Mushroom Ragu with Spaghetti

If you're trying to eat less meat, this is the ideal entry-level meal. It tastes so rich and flavoursome that you won't miss the meat. Even my husband, a devout carnivore, is a convert! It also tastes even better the next day and is equally good over a baked sweet potato or as a base for a vegan shepherd's pie. The combined ingredients contribute eight of your thirty different plants per week, which studies have shown is optimal for gut health. Lentil ragu freezes particularly well, so I often batch-cook it, ready for busy weeknights.

Serves 4

2 tbsp olive oil

1 small onion, diced

3 garlic cloves, chopped

1 carrot, diced

1 celery stick, diced

250g mushrooms, finely chopped

1 bay leaf

400g tin chopped tomatoes

1 tbsp tomato purée

a pinch of dried chilli flakes

250ml vegetable stock

400g can green lentils, drained and rinsed

300g whole-wheat spaghetti

2 tbsp chopped parsley

salt and ground black pepper

Parmesan or vegan cheese, to serve

Heat the oil in a heavy-based saucepan over a medium heat. Add the onion, garlic, carrot and celery and cook for 10 minutes or until the onions are translucent.

Add the mushrooms and cook for 5–10 minutes until soft.

Add the bay leaf, chopped tomatoes, tomato purée, chilli flakes, vegetable stock and lentils, then bring to the boil. Reduce the heat and simmer, covered, for 20 minutes. Season with salt and pepper to taste.

Cook the pasta in a saucepan of boiling water for 8 minutes or according to the pack instructions, drain and return to the pan then stir in the lentil ragu. Sprinkle with the parsley, remove the bay leaf and serve with freshly grated Parmesan.

Cajun Salmon with Mango and Avocado Salsa

I'm always looking for new ways to incorporate salmon into weekday meals, and I came up with this recipe when we had some leftover fajita spice mix. Now I make it more often than the fajitas, but such is the evolution of recipes.

The sweet and tangy salsa complements the warm spiced salmon and adds vibrant colour to the plate. Mangoes are loaded with beta-carotene and vitamin C, which help to fight free-radical damage. Add a side of your favourite grain to round off the meal – I often use microwaveable pouches for ease and speed.

Serves 4

4 salmon fillets (or one large 500g fillet)

1 tbsp olive oil

your grain of choice, cooked, to serve

For the Cajun spice mix:

(I often make double or triple the quantity and store it in an airtight jar for future use)

1 tsp ground cumin

½ tsp paprika

½ tsp dried oregano

½ tsp dried thyme

1 tsp garlic powder or 1 garlic clove, crushed

½ tsp chilli powder

1 tsp sea salt

For the mango and avocado salsa:

2 ripe avocados, diced

2 large mangoes, diced

½ small red onion, diced

½ red chilli, deseeded and finely chopped

juice of 1 lime, plus 1 lime cut into quarters

1 tbsp chopped coriander leaves

salt and pepper

Preheat the oven to 200°C (180°C fan oven) Gas 6 and line a baking tray with foil. Combine the Cajun spice mix ingredients in a small bowl.

Pat the salmon dry with kitchen paper and massage with the olive oil, then sprinkle the spice mix over the surface.

Put the salmon, skin-side down, on the prepared baking tray and bake for 12–15 minutes until cooked through and the flesh flakes easily.

While your salmon is cooking, combine the salsa ingredients in a bowl. Serve alongside the salmon, with lime wedges and your favourite grain.

Cajun Cauliflower

If you'd like to make a vegan version of the above recipe, I suggest using cauliflower. The Cajun spice mix above should be adequate for one whole cauliflower that has been separated into florets. Coat with oil and the spice mix and bake at 220°C (200°C fan oven) Gas 7 for 20 minutes or until crispy.

Spaghetti with Walnut Pesto, Courgette and Peas

This is pesto pasta the SkinFood way. Walnut pesto is quick and easy to make, and it goes with everything, from salads to soups, or as a spread in a sandwich. Walnuts have a richer nutrient profile than pine nuts and are full of skin-loving omega-3. They are also more economical too. If you are allergic to walnuts, stick to the traditional version (pine nuts are in fact a seed). You'll need quite a bit of olive oil for this recipe, not only to create a rich flavour but also to provide healthy fats. This dish is great alone or alongside some simply grilled chicken, spread on tomato and ricotta toast (page 289), or drizzled onto a bowl of Tuscan bean soup (page 303).

Serves 2

150g whole-wheat spaghetti

1 courgette, diced

100g frozen peas

freshly grated Parmesan, to serve

For the pesto:

45g walnuts

2 garlic cloves, roughly chopped

2 × 30g packs of basil

½ tsp salt

160ml extra-virgin olive oil, plus a little extra to finish

50g freshly grated Parmesan cheese

ground black pepper

Begin by making the pesto. Put the walnuts and garlic in a food processer and chop coarsely. Add the basil leaves, salt and black pepper to taste, and blend until you start to form a paste. Add the olive oil in batches, pulsing to combine until completely blended.

Add the grated Parmesan and blend for approximately 1 minute to combine. Store in a clean, airtight jar. A thin layer of olive oil on the top keeps it fresh and green, allowing it to keep in the fridge for up to 2 weeks.

Cook the spaghetti in a saucepan of boiling water according to the pack instructions. Five minutes before the end of cooking, add the courgette and peas.

Drain in a colander and stir through 2–3 tbsp of the walnut pesto to taste (or more if you prefer). Serve with plenty of grated Parmesan.

Seared Fish with Fennel, Orange and Olives

White fish is an excellent source of complete protein, providing all the amino acids needed for building healthy skin and hair. You can buy fresh or frozen, either is fine, but please do seek out sustainable options where possible. Fennel and orange combine to make a tart and sweet salad, which is one of my go-tos, particularly in the summer. Fennel has an impressive nutrient profile, containing over 80 different antioxidants, such as quercetin and rosmarinic acid, which protect against free-radical damage and inflammation. Orange is abundant in vitamin C, of course, and olives are rich in skin-smoothing vitamin E.

Serves 4

2 oranges

2 tbsp pitted black olives

2 fennel bulbs, thinly sliced

2 tbsp olive oil, plus 1 tbsp for frying

juice of ½ orange

2 tbsp pine nuts (optional), toasted (see tip below)

4 white fish fillets of your choice

salt and ground black pepper

cooked whole grain of choice (such as whole-wheat couscous or brown rice), to serve

Using a sharp knife, cut off the top and bottom of the oranges and then cut off the skin and pith from top to bottom. Slice the flesh thinly into rings. Put the olives, fennel and orange in a bowl. (Or, if you are serving this dish to guests, you can make it look extra pretty by arranging the orange and fennel slices on a serving plate and sprinkling over the olives.)

Put the 2 tbsp olive oil in a small bowl and add the orange juice. Season with salt and pepper to taste, and mix well. Pour over the fennel-mixture ingredients. Top with toasted pine nuts for added crunch (if using).

Pat the fish fillets dry with kitchen paper and season with salt and pepper. Heat the 1 tbsp olive oil in a frying pan over a medium-high heat. Once the oil is hot, add the fish (skin-side down if it's skin-on), and sear until crispy on one side, then flip and continue cooking until cooked through and the flesh flakes easily.

Serve with the side salad and a whole grain of your choice. This would also be great with Jewelled Couscous (page 329), or Walnut Pesto Spaghetti (page 325).

Pine nuts
Lightly toast pine nuts in a dry pan over a medium-low heat until golden. Watch carefully, as they can burn easily.

Butternut Chickpea and Apricot Tagine with Jewelled Couscous

Golden butternut squash is an abundant source of skin-loving nutrients. It is rich in three different carotenoids that are converted to vitamin A, which is essential for skin repair and protection against ageing. It also contains B vitamins and plenty of vitamin C, as well as lots of fibre to keep gut bacteria happy. Chickpeas are an excellent source of protein, and the turmeric-infused jewelled couscous adds glow-boosting essential fats.

You could easily double this recipe if you're entertaining or batch-cooking for the rest of the week. Or you can make a lovely gluten-free version by choosing a different grain in place of couscous, such as quinoa or brown rice.

Serves 4–6

1 tbsp olive oil

1 red onion, sliced

2 garlic cloves, chopped

2 tsp ground turmeric

2 tsp ground cumin

2 tsp sweet paprika

300g butternut squash, cubed (roughly ½ whole squash)

1 tbsp harissa paste

1 tbsp tomato purée

400ml vegetable stock

2 × 400g tins chickpeas, drained and rinsed

40g dried apricots, sliced

2 tbsp coriander leaves

salt and ground black pepper

For the jewelled couscous:

200g wholegrain couscous

1 tsp ground turmeric

250ml boiling vegetable stock

40g flaked almonds

80g pomegranate seeds

Heat the oil in a heavy-based saucepan over a medium heat. Add the onion, garlic and a pinch of salt to the pan and cook for 5–6 minutes to allow the onion to caramelise.

Add the turmeric, sweet paprika and cumin, and cook for 1–2 minutes until they become fragrant, and then add the butternut squash cubes and cook for 2–3 minutes until softened.

Add the harissa paste and tomato purée, then the stock, chickpeas and apricots. Bring to the boil then reduce the heat, cover and cook over a medium heat for 40 minutes. Season to taste with salt and pepper.

To make the couscous, put the couscous in a large bowl. Stir the turmeric into the boiling vegetable stock and then pour it over the couscous. Leave to soak for 5–10 minutes until fluffy.

Stir in the nuts and pomegranate seeds. Serve by spooning the tagine over the couscous and topping with coriander leaves.

Vegan Chilli-Loaded Sweet Potatoes

I first developed this recipe as part of my Nutrition Science coursework and have been enjoying it ever since. Beans are one of my top skin foods, as they are rich in a range of minerals and vitamins as well as protein and fibre. I've used them in this recipe to create a vegan version of a versatile family favourite. This chilli is great over baked potatoes, a bowl of brown rice or even over some corn tortillas for nutrition-boosted nachos.

Serves 4–6

4 even-sized sweet potatoes

2 tbsp olive oil

1 onion, sliced

2 carrots, diced

2 celery sticks, diced

1 red pepper, deseeded and chopped

2 garlic cloves, chopped

2 tsp ground cumin

1 tsp chilli powder, or to taste

2 tsp smoked paprika

1 tsp dried oregano (optional)

2 × 400g tins chopped tomatoes

400g tin black beans, drained and rinsed

400g tin kidney beans, drained and rinsed

salt and ground black pepper

To serve:

250g yoghurt of choice

1 avocado, sliced

50g cheese of your choice, grated

Preheat the oven to 200°C (180°C fan oven) Gas 6 and bake the sweet potatoes for 45 minutes or until soft when squeezed with a cloth.

Heat the oil in a large saucepan over a medium heat. Add the onion, carrots, celery and red pepper, and season with a pinch of salt. Stir well and cook for 7–10 minutes until soft.

Add the garlic, cumin, chilli powder, smoked paprika and oregano (if using) and cook for 1 minute until fragrant.

Add the chopped tomatoes, black beans and kidney beans, and stir well. Bring to the boil then reduce the heat to a gentle simmer for 30 minutes, covered.

Once the chilli is cooked, taste and add salt and pepper to taste as required. If you prefer a thicker consistency, you can also finish by blending it partly using an immersion blender.

Serve over the baked sweet potatoes with a generous helping of the yoghurt, avocado and cheese.

Supercharged Roasted Tofu, Sweet Potato and Broccoli Bake

I love one-pan cooking. You can throw all your ingredients in the oven and out comes something so much more delicious than the sum of its parts. Broccoli is the surprising star of this recipe. As part of the brassica family, it contains sulforaphane, which powerfully reduces inflammation and oxidative stress. Early research has also shown that it can have an anti-inflammatory effect on skin conditions such as eczema and psoriasis, as well as protecting against ageing. But there is an important trick when cooking with broccoli: you should cut it and leave it for 10–15 minutes before heating. This helps to boost the sulforaphane levels for maximum benefits. The same goes for onions and garlic, but I'm usually just too impatient to do this every time!

Serves 2

300g block of tofu, drained and rinsed, and cut into cubes

1 head of broccoli, broken into florets

2 sweet potatoes, roughly chopped

1 pepper (red or yellow), deseeded and cut into chunks

1 red onion, cut into chunks

2 tbsp sunflower seeds

cooked grain (optional), to serve

For the dressing:

juice of 1 lime

1 tbsp maple syrup or honey

1 tbsp soy sauce

1 tsp miso paste

2 tbsp avocado or olive oil

2 garlic cloves, grated

½ tsp dried chilli flakes (optional)

Preheat the oven to 220°C (200°C fan oven) Gas 7 and line a baking tray with baking paper. Put the dressing ingredients in a small bowl and stir to combine.

Spread the tofu, broccoli, sweet potatoes, pepper and red onion on the prepared baking tray and drizzle over your dressing, ensuring that all the ingredients are well coated. Cook in the oven for 30 minutes.

Sprinkle over the sunflower seeds and cook for a further 5–10 minutes until cooked through and the seeds are golden. Enjoy on its own or serve it over your favourite grain. This also makes an excellent portable lunch.

The Ultimate Skin Fuel Salad

We all need a recipe we can turn to when we want to look and feel our best in advance of a big event. This salad ticks all the boxes and contains some of my favourite skin foods topped with a probiotic-rich tangy miso dressing. It's both filling and flavoursome as well as being gorgeously good for you.

If you're short on time, feel free to use pre-cooked, vacuum-packed salmon fillets – although try to avoid anything honey-glazed, as it tends to be higher in refined sugar. You could just as easily replace the salmon with spiced chickpeas (page 334), however, or crispy tofu (page 315) if you eat a plant-based diet.

Serves 2
75g baby spinach
40g cashew nuts

100g cherry tomatoes, halved

1 avocado, flesh sliced

½ cucumber, cut into chunks

2 pre-cooked salmon fillets

200g cooked grain of choice, cooled

For the dressing:

1 tbsp miso paste

juice of 1 lime

1 tsp honey

0.5cm fresh ginger, peeled and grated, or ½ tsp ginger paste

½ tsp grated garlic or ½ garlic clove, crushed

1 tbsp olive or avocado oil

Put the spinach, nuts, tomatoes, avocado and cucumber in a large serving bowl. Gently flake apart the salmon fillets and add them to the salad, along with the cooked and cooled grains.

Put the dressing ingredients in a small bowl and whisk together until combined.

Pour half the dressing over the salad and toss together using salad tongs. There should be enough dressing left over for 2 further servings; you can store this in the fridge in a sealed jar for 4 days.

Spiced Chickpea Salad with Yoghurt

This is the sort of food you want to share with friends. Warm spiced chickpeas are the star of this dish and I adore them for their versatility and punch of nutrients. I first made a Middle Eastern spiced chickpea salad many years ago and as much as I loved the flavours, I wanted to make my own version with

Indian spices. I like to serve this topped with probiotic yoghurt and some whole-wheat pittas to scoop up the delicious juices, but it also goes perfectly with the Harissa-Spiced Turkey Burgers on page 321.

Serves 2 as a main or 4 as a starter

½ cucumber, cut into 2cm cubes

200g cherry tomatoes, quartered

1 small red onion, finely diced

1 red pepper, deseeded and cut into 2cm cubes

2 tbsp olive oil

juice of ½ lemon

200g yoghurt of choice

1 tsp harissa paste (optional)

1 garlic clove, grated

0.5cm fresh ginger, peeled and grated, or ½ tsp ginger paste

1 tsp ground cumin

1 tsp ground coriander

½ tsp chilli powder

½ tsp ground turmeric

400g tin chickpeas, drained and rinsed

salt and ground black pepper

a handful of coriander leaves

warm whole-wheat bread, chapatti or pitta, to serve

Put the cucumber, cherry tomatoes, red onion and red pepper in a large bowl. Season with salt and pepper to taste and stir in 1 tbsp of the olive oil and the lemon juice.

In a small bowl, mix the yoghurt with the harissa paste (if using).

Heat the remaining oil in a frying pan over a medium heat, add the garlic, ginger, cumin, coriander, chilli powder and turmeric,

and heat for a few minutes until fragrant. Add the chickpeas to the
pan and cook for 10 minutes until well coated with the spices and
heated through.

Place the salad mixture on a flat serving dish, layer the warm
chickpeas on top, then drizzle over the yoghurt. Top with coriander
and serve with warm bread.

Snacks and desserts

I recommend a small snack mid-morning and mid-afternoon
to help stabilise blood sugar levels and keep cravings at bay. To
store snacks, I use an airtight container with two compartments
(such as one with nuts and another with fruit), which helps to
remind me to keep my snacks balanced. My favourite go-to
snacks are usually very simple:

- Small handful of nuts (cashew nuts/almonds/pistachio
  nuts/pecan nuts/hazelnuts) and a piece of fruit or a
  handful of berries
- Small pot of yoghurt with seeds and fruit
- Oatcakes and carrot sticks with hummus
- Boiled egg and sliced red pepper
- Avocado mashed onto brown rice cakes
- Sliced apple and nut or seed butter
- Roasted chickpeas and sliced cucumber
- Few squares of dark chocolate, pear and a
  few almonds
- Dried apricots and pecan nuts

For dessert, I love a few squares of dark chocolate after dinner, and there are so many to choose from now. I like mine with hazelnuts or almonds, but there are extremely good dairy- and nut-free versions available. I've talked before about cocoa percentages (page 127) so I won't go into too much detail here, but chocolate is most certainly not off the menu.

Let's now dive into my snack and dessert recipes to satisfy all of your sweet or salty cravings!

Beautifully Bright Beetroot Hummus with Crudités

Hummus makes the perfect snack, as it's full of fibre, vitamins and good fats from the olive oil. I prefer to make my own, as the oil used in store-bought varieties is usually made with vegetable oil, so you might lose the benefits of healthy fats. I've added beetroot to this recipe for an extra boost, as it contains B vitamins and vitamin C, and it can also improve blood circulation. There are many reasons to make this dip, but my favourite has to be the colour: it is unashamedly fuchsia pink.

Makes 6 servings

400g tin chickpeas, drained and rinsed

250g cooked beetroot

juice of 1 lemon

2 garlic cloves

2 tbsp tahini

4 tbsp olive oil

½ tsp ground cumin

salt and ground black pepper

oatcakes and crudités, such as carrots, cucumber, celery, peppers and sugar snap peas, to serve

Put all the ingredients, except the olive oil, in a food processor and blend until smooth.

Slowly add the olive oil in small batches, blending after each addition. Season to taste with salt and pepper. Enjoy with oatcakes and crudités.

Roasted Spiced Nuts

As I'm sure you've realised, nuts are one of my top skin foods and I encourage you to have them daily if you can. Although raw unsalted nuts are best, it is always good to have a little variety. You can use whatever combination of nuts you like to make this, but I love walnuts, cashew nuts and almonds.

Makes 8–10 servings
2 tbsp olive oil
½ tsp sea salt
1 tsp ground cumin
1 tsp sweet paprika
½ tsp chilli powder
300g mixed nuts
ground black pepper

Preheat the oven to 200°C (180°C fan oven) Gas 6 and line a baking sheet with baking paper. Mix the oil, salt and spices together in a bowl.

Add the nuts to the bowl and season with a generous grind of black pepper. Stir to ensure that they are well coated in the spiced oil.

Spread the nuts in a single layer on the prepared baking sheet and roast for 15 minutes, turning them over halfway. Leave to cool completely before storing them in an airtight container for up to 1 week.

Gorgeous Guacamole

There is nothing like freshly made guacamole. This makes four generous servings, and I like to add it to Chilli-Loaded Sweet Potatoes (page 330) or enjoy it as a dip with corn tortilla crackers. In the summer, my family gets through bowlfuls of this, and it's a huge crowd pleaser.

Serves 4

3 ripe avocados

2 spring onions, finely diced

1 tomato, finely diced

3 tbsp chopped coriander leaves

1 garlic clove, crushed

1 tbsp jalapeño peppers from a jar (or one fresh)

Tabasco sauce, to taste

juice of 1 lime

salt and ground black pepper

Scoop out the avocado flesh into a mixing bowl and mash with a fork or potato masher (I prefer the latter when I am making large quantities).

Add the spring onions, tomato, coriander leaves, garlic and jalapeño pepper to the bowl and mix well to combine. Season to taste with salt, pepper, Tabasco sauce and lime juice.

Roasted Red Pepper and Walnut Dip

I am always looking at ways to incorporate healthy fats into recipes, and this speedy take on the classic Middle Eastern *Muhammara* fits the bill perfectly. Not only is it loaded with vitamin-packed red peppers, but it also has healthy fats from both the olive oil and walnuts.

Serves 6

200g roasted red peppers from a jar (or three oven-roasted red peppers)

60g walnuts

½ tsp dried chilli flakes

1 garlic clove

½ tsp ground cumin

juice of ½ lemon

3 tbsp olive oil

salt and ground black pepper

whole-wheat pitta chips or freshly cut vegetables, to serve

Put all the ingredients in a blender or food processor and combine until smooth. Season to taste with salt and pepper. Serve with whole-wheat pitta.

The APPLE Study Muffins

I devised these moist and sweet muffins to celebrate our research project, the APPLE (Asking People with Psoriasis about Lifestyle and Eating) Study – so, of course, it had to be an apple-based recipe but elevated with skin-boosting ingredients.

This research project is the first to take a deep dive into the relationship between nutrition and psoriasis. Wholesome and fruit-filled, these muffins can be stored in an airtight container for 2–3 days after baking. If you'd like to make this recipe vegan, you can replace the eggs with flaxseeds instead.

Makes 12 muffins

oil, for greasing

200g whole-wheat flour (self-raising) or gluten-free flour

1½ tsp baking powder

½ tsp bicarbonate of soda

2 tsp ground cinnamon

½ tsp salt

2 apples, diced or grated

80ml olive oil

100ml honey or maple syrup

2 eggs (or 2 flax eggs: 2 tbsp ground flaxseed and 2½ tbsp water mixed and left to stand for 10 minutes)

120g pouch of apple/banana purée (I get mine from the baby food section)

120ml yoghurt of your choice

1 tsp vanilla extract

Preheat the oven to 200°C (180°C fan oven) Gas 6 and line a 12-cup muffin tray with muffin cases, then grease the cases (I use an oil spray). Sift the flour, baking powder, bicarbonate of soda, cinnamon and salt into a large mixing bowl.

Add the apples and stir to bring the mixture together.

In a separate bowl, whisk together the oil and honey, and then beat in the eggs or flax eggs.

Add the apple purée to the egg mixture followed by the yoghurt and vanilla. Mix well, then pour into the large mixing bowl with the dry ingredients and stir together until combined. The mixture won't be completely smooth because of the apple, but try to break down as many lumps as possible.

Divide evenly among the muffin cases and bake for 20–25 minutes or until a skewer inserted into the centre comes out clean. Leave to cool completely. These muffins will keep for up to 2 days in an airtight container and they also freeze well.

Avocado, Coconut and Lime Ice Cream

I had my first taste of this unbelievably good combination of flavours while on holiday in Croatia. I really did not expect it to be as tasty as it was. I couldn't wait to get home and try to make it myself and, although not exactly the same, this is a very close approximation. There are only five ingredients to this and, while it needs a bit of prep, it is so quick to make.

Serves 6

2 ripe avocados
1 ripe banana, chopped into chunks
4 tbsp maple syrup or honey
400ml tin full-fat coconut milk
juice and zest of ½ lime

Chill a 20cm loaf pan in the fridge for 30 minutes. Meanwhile, scoop out the avocado flesh and pop it into a blender or food processor.

Add the banana, maple syrup, coconut milk and lime zest and juice. Blend on a high speed, scraping down the edges of the blender, until you have a very smooth consistency. Place the mixture in the chilled loaf pan and spread evenly. Freeze for at least 6 hours but preferably overnight.

Allow the ice cream to soften for a good 10–15 minutes before serving.

Tips

- This recipe works even better if you freeze the avocados and banana chunks ahead of time before blending.
- Serve the ice cream with melted dark chocolate poured over, for a delicious treat. To melt chocolate, put it in a heatproof bowl over a pan of gently simmering water, making sure the base of the bowl doesn't touch the water. Leave until melted, stirring occasionally.

Chocolate, Banana and Buckwheat Loaf

Fudgy and rich, this banana bread never lasts long in my house, as it makes the perfect snack or breakfast on the go. Although I love a traditional banana bread, my aim with this recipe was to boost nutrients without compromising on flavour and texture, so I really hope you enjoy it.

I've used buckwheat flour, as it is a naturally gluten-free whole grain and has a nutty flavour that works really well with bananas and chocolate. You could always replace it with plain whole-wheat or other gluten-free flour.

Makes 1 loaf

75ml olive oil or melted coconut oil, plus extra for greasing

60ml milk of choice

3 bananas, very ripe and mashed with a fork

2 eggs

1 tsp vanilla extract

220g buckwheat flour

60g brown sugar

½ tsp ground cinnamon

½ tsp salt

½ tsp bicarbonate of soda

1 tsp baking powder

100g dark chocolate chips

Preheat the oven to 200°C (180°C fan oven) Gas 6 and line a 23 × 13cm loaf pan with baking paper then grease the paper well.

Pour the oil and milk into a large mixing bowl and whisk together. Add the mashed bananas, eggs and vanilla and combine well.

In a separate bowl sift together the flour, sugar, cinnamon, salt, bicarbonate of soda and baking powder.

Pour the wet ingredient mix into the bowl with the dry ingredients and stir until combined. Add the chocolate chips, and stir to ensure that they are evenly distributed.

Spread the mix into the prepared loaf pan and bake in the oven for 40 minutes until a skewer inserted into the centre comes out clean. Leave in the pan on a wire rack to cool, then turn out and leave to cool completely before slicing.

SkinFood Chocolate Cherry Brownies

Just one bite of these moist, decadent brownies is all you'll need to be convinced that nutritious foods can be delicious too. This is the ultimate SkinFood recipe, and one that I urge you to try. As you'll see from the cover of this book, I have a little bit of an obsession with cherries, as they have the most extraordinary antioxidant profile, which is in part due to their deep purple colour. These brownies are rich in fibre, thanks to gut-loving dates, and dark chocolate is good for the skin too!

Makes 12 squares

6 Medjool dates

75ml olive oil or rapeseed oil

70g sugar

1 tbsp honey

60g plain whole-wheat flour

30g cocoa powder

a pinch of salt

3 eggs, beaten

1 tsp vanilla extract

150g pitted cherries (fresh or frozen), chopped

50g chocolate chips

30g sliced almonds

Preheat the oven to 170°C (150°C fan oven) Gas 3.

Remove the seeds from the Medjool dates, place them in a large bowl, and cover with boiling water so that they soak for 20 minutes. Meanwhile, warm the oil, sugar and honey in a pan until combined and liquid.

In a separate bowl mix together the flour, cocoa powder and salt. Once the dates have finished soaking, place them in a food processer along with two tablespoons of the soaking liquid and blend to form a smooth paste. Stir this paste into your dry ingredients, and add the beaten eggs, vanilla, as well as the warmed sugar, oil and honey and stir well to combine. Finally add the cherries, chocolate chips and almonds and stir again until the ingredients are evenly distributed.

Pour the mixture into a lined, 20cm square baking tin and bake for 30 minutes until moist and fudgy. Allow to cool before cutting into squares.

Gut-Loving Pear, Blackberry and Ginger Crumble

This is a lighter and gut-loving version of the classic English crumble. It makes for a delicious dessert as well as a warming breakfast. I still enjoy a traditional crumble, but when I want something more nourishing, this fits the bill. Ginger helps to soothe digestion and reduce bloating, while flaxseeds add nuttiness to the crumble topping, and blackberries are an excellent source of vitamin C.

Serves 4

50g plain whole-wheat flour

25g rolled (porridge) oats

2 tbsp ground flaxseeds

25g soft brown sugar

½ tsp ground cinnamon

30g butter or spread of choice

4 ripe pears, peeled and roughly cubed

150g blackberries

2 tsp freshly grated ginger

yoghurt, to serve

Preheat the oven to 200°C (180°C fan oven) Gas 6. Put the flour, oats, flaxseeds, sugar, cinnamon in a bowl and rub together with the butter until coarse breadcrumbs begin to form.

Put the pears in an ovenproof dish along with the blackberries, add the grated ginger and mix to combine. Spoon the crumble mixture over the fruit to form an even layer.

Bake for 20–25 minutes until the top is golden and the fruit is soft. Serve with your favourite yoghurt.

Rose and Ashwagandha Beauty Sleep Latte

As we learned in Chapter 7, sleep is a vital part of skin health, and a lack of adequate sleep can show up in our skin. This beautifully pink latte has been devised to help you drift off at night a little more easily. It contains ashwagandha, which has been shown in studies to support sleep and reduce anxiety (see page 220).

It's important that you start with a low dose of half a teaspoon, but you can slowly increase your intake to up to one teaspoon, if it suits you. As with any supplements, check with your doctor before introducing it into your diet to make sure it doesn't interact with any existing medications and omit if you are pregnant or breastfeeding.

A little beetroot powder gives this latte its gorgeous colour and also adds an extra hit of antioxidants.

Serves 1

250ml milk of choice, unsweetened

½ tsp vanilla extract

½ tsp ashwagandha powder, no more than 300μg

a pinch of beetroot powder

½ tsp rosewater

Warm the milk in a small saucepan over a medium heat. Add the vanilla, beetroot powder, rosewater and ashwagandha powder and stir until fully combined.

Enjoy warm, in your favourite mug, cosied up in bed.

Chapter summary

- Before making any changes to your diet, preparation is key – think about why you want to make these changes and how you want to put them into practice.
- Check your kitchen to see what you do have, before stocking up with SkinFood essentials.
- The foundation for your meals throughout the day is GLOW (see page 279), the aim is to eat these components throughout the day rather than at every single meal.
- Be kind to yourself; this isn't a diet, it's a plan to suit your needs.
- There is no need for deprivation; enjoy your meals and the pleasure of eating good food.

Final Words

Our skin is the unique reflection of our internal health and our external world. How we eat, sleep, drink and care for it shows, which is precisely why I developed the 4-Step Skin Solution. Through research and years spent treating patients, I have realised that we need to start taking a more holistic approach to skincare and to go deeper than just the products that we put on our skin or the prescriptions we take, but also to consider how our diet and our mental well-being might be affecting our appearance.

Through the latest research, cutting-edge nutritional insight and stories from the clinic that I've shared over the course of this book, you've seen the incredible way that our skin can be restored to health with a combination of all four steps of these steps. It is because of my patients and being able to witness their skin transformations that I was motivated to write this book, as I wanted to demystify the path to healthy skin and to make it achievable for all.

I hope you're feeling motivated and eager to incorporate my advice to improve your skin, but the best bit is that you're going to gain so much more than a beautiful complexion in the process: you'll be nourishing your mind and body – and this is the real key to long-term health and happiness.

Resources

For further information on common skin conditions:
  skinsupport.org.uk
  www.skinhealthinfo.org.uk
  www.britishskinfoundation.org.uk

For further information on nutrition:
  www.nhs.uk/conditions/vitamins-and-minerals
  www.bda.uk.com/food-health/food-facts/all-food-fact-sheets

For information on how to find a specialist:
  You can find a dietitian via the British Dietetic Association: www.bda.uk.com/find-a-dietitian
  You can find a therapist through the UKCP or BACP: www.psychotherapy.org.uk/find-a-therapist and www.bacp.co.uk/about-therapy/using-our-therapist-directory
  You can find an allergy specialist through the BSACI: www.bsaci.org/workforce/find-a-clinic

Cosmetic treatments

You can find certified practitioners for cosmetic and laser treatments on the register at Joint Council of Cosmetic Practitioners. Website: jccp.org.uk

The Dermatology Life Quality Index

You can try this test yourself, but please remember to share your scores with your care provider to help direct treatment: www. cardiff.ac.uk/medicine/resources/quality-of-life-questionnaires/ dermatology-life-quality-index

Disordered eating

If you feel that you might be experiencing a form of disordered eating, please do discuss this with a qualified health professional. The following websites may also be useful resources:

www.beateatingdisorders.org.uk

www.mind.org.uk/information-support/ types-of-mental-health-problems/eating-problems

Eczema

National Eczema Society: www.eczema.org.

To learn more about habit reversal: https://www.atopicskin-disease.com/

Download a trigger diary: https://www.allergyuk.org/ resources/food-and-symptoms-diary/

Food allergies

For information on food allergies and allergy testing: www. allergyuk.org

Gratitude journaling
Positive affirmation cards have been produced by the Real Skin
Club: www.realskinclub.com

Mind–body connection
See the National Eczema Society for more about the mind–body
connection: https://eczema.org/blog/the-mind-body-connection
   Psychodermatology is a unique field within dermatology that
addresses the mind–skin connection: www.psychodermatology.
co.uk/information

Mindfulness
The British Association of Dermatologists has devoted an entire
web page to mindfulness meditation that features five specific
guided meditations for people living with skin conditions
such as eczema and psoriasis. Website: skinsupport.org.uk/
support-materials/meditation-mindfulness.

Medical treatments
To find out more about treatments mentioned in this book visit:
https://www.bad.org.uk/patient-information-leaflets

Psoriasis
For further information and advice about psoriasis, visit the
Psoriasis Association: www.psoriasis-association.org.uk/
   Another charity that supports people with psoriasis and pso-
riatic arthritis is the Psoriasis and Psoriatic Arthritis Alliance:
www.papaa.org/
   To take part in our research at King's College London visit:
www.dietandpsoriasisproject-apple.com
   To watch a video on how to treat psoriasis in the scalp from

the team at Guy's and St Thomas' NHS Trust visit: www.you-tube.com/watch?v=hMUPuqt-khY

Rosacea

You can find out more about rosacea via the National Rosacea Society: www.rosacea.org/patients/materials/rosacea-diary-booklet

Acknowledgements

They say that 'a journey of a thousand miles starts with a single step' and writing this book has certainly been quite the journey. I would not have been able to take the first step, or the many others that followed, without the love and support of my husband, James. His unwavering faith has made this book possible, and I am eternally grateful for the many hats he has worn throughout the process – including editor, therapist, human thesaurus – and of course for taking such good care of our beloved boys, Oscar, Rafferty and Atticus, so that I could spend weekends and evenings writing. I am so sorry to have missed out on time with my boys, but I hope this book will make them proud one day. I owe so much to my loving family, my mother, brother Ben and sister-in-law Ella, for always checking in, advising and guiding as I navigated this uncharted territory.

I am hugely indebted to my editor, Bernadette Marron, at Little, Brown for all her hard work, helping to refine the manuscript and make it digestible, and for putting up with my constantly evolving deadlines as I edited and re-edited the text at the very last moment. It is now a book I feel proud of and this is thanks to your efforts. Richard Pike, my literary agent at C&W, has been indispensable throughout the process, and I'd like to thank him for his calm guidance and extraordinary patience. Thank you also to Ellen Rockell for the unmistakable cherry cover design and to Elke Desanghere and Matthew Crossey at Little, Brown. Susan Watt provided a measured review of the early manuscript, helping to make the science readable and relevant. In addition, Anne Wright and Harriet Smith forensically examined specific chapters to ensure their dietetic robustness. Their edits were invaluable in improving the quality of the final text.

This book would not have been published without an initial introduction from Ian Marber, who was kind enough to send the original proposal to his editor, I am indebted to you for this.

I thank my colleagues in the department of nutritional sciences, King's College London who have allowed research in nutritional dermatology to flourish, as well as the Psoriasis Association for supporting our research. My mentors in dermatology have given me the confidence to explore new research avenues and include Professor Christopher Griffiths, and Professor Edel O'Toole.

Finally, I thank the patients I have seen over the years. I have learned more from you than I could possibly explain in words; your questions on the links between nutrition and the skin set me on this path, and my sincerest hope is that by learning from your experiences, this book can go on to help many others.

References

INTRODUCTION

1. Source: All Party Parliamentary Group on Skin Report, 2020

I THE FUNDAMENTALS: SKIN SCHOOL

1. Maruthappu T, Hader Z (2021). A characteristic rash caused by Shiitake mushrooms - An emerging concern? *Clin Case Rep.* May 5;9(6):e04181
2. Maruthappu T, Posafalvi A, Castelletti S, Delaney PJ, Syrris P, O'Toole EA, Green KJ, Elliott PM, Lambiase PD, Tinker A, McKenna WJ, Kelsell DP. (2019). Loss-of-function desmoplakin I and II mutations underlie dominant arrhythmogenic cardiomyopathy with a hair and skin phenotype. *Br J Dermatol.* 2019 May;180(5):1114-1122.
3. Maruthappu T, Taylor M. Acne and rosacea in skin of colour (2022). *Clin Exp Dermatol.* Feb;47(2):259-263.
4. Christensen K, Thinggaard M, McGue M, Rexbye H, Hjelmborg JV, Aviv A, Gunn D, van der Ouderaa F, Vaupel JW (2009). Perceived age as clinically useful biomarker of ageing: cohort study. *BMJ.* Dec 10;339
5. Krutmann J, Bouloc A, Sore G, Bernard BA, Passeron T. The skin aging exposome (2017). *J Dermatol Sci.* Mar;85(3):152-161

6. Kim HS. Microbiota in Rosacea (2020). *Am J Clin Dermatol.* Sep;21(Suppl 1):25-35

7. Sandilands A, Sutherland C, Irvine AD, McLean WH (2009). Filaggrin in the frontline: role in skin barrier function and disease. *J Cell Sci.* May 1;122

2 NUTRIENTS THAT NOURISH, FROM A TO ZINC

1. Berry, S.E., Valdes, A.M., Drew, D.A. et al. Human postprandial responses to food and potential for precision nutrition. *Nat Med* 26, 964–973 (2020)

2. Source: Glycemicindex.com

3. Nguyen HP, Katta R. Sugar Sag: Glycation and the Role of Diet in Aging Skin (2015). *Skin Therapy Lett.* Nov;20(6):1-5

4. Kendall AC, Pilkington SM, Murphy SA, Del Carratore F, Sunarwidhi AL, Kiezel-Tsugunova M, Urquhart P, Watson REB, Breitling R, Rhodes LE, Nicolaou A. Dynamics of the human skin mediator lipidome in response to dietary ω-3 fatty acid supplementation (2019). *FASEB J.* Nov;33(11):13014-13027

5. Source: https://www.bda.uk.com/resource/omega-3.html

6. Mostafa WZ, Hegazy RA. Vitamin D and the skin: Focus on a complex relationship: A review(2015). *J Adv Res.* Nov;6(6):793-804

7. Passeron T, Bouillon R, Callender V, Cestari T, Diepgen TL, Green AC, van der Pols JC, Bernard BA, Ly F, Bernerd F, Marrot L, Nielsen M, Verschoore M, Jablonski NG, Young AR. Sunscreen photoprotection and vitamin D status (2019). *Br J Dermatol.* Nov;181(5):916-931

8. Mulligan GB, Licata A. Taking vitamin D with the largest meal improves absorption and results in higher serum levels of 25-hydroxyvitamin D (2010). *J Bone Miner Res.* Apr;25(4):928-30

9. Keen MA, Hassan I. Vitamin E in dermatology (2016). *Indian Dermatol Online* J. Jul-Aug;7(4):311-5

10. Chen AC, Martin AJ, Choy B, Fernández-Peñas P, Dalziell RA, McKenzie CA, Scolyer RA, Dhillon HM, Vardy JL, Kricker A, St George G, Chinniah N, Halliday GM, Damian DL. A Phase 3 Randomized Trial of Nicotinamide for Skin-Cancer Chemoprevention(2015). *N Engl J Med.* Oct 22;373(17):1618-26

11. Barbosa E, Faintuch J, Machado Moreira EA, Gonçalves da
    Silva VR, Lopes Pereima MJ, Martins Fagundes RL, Filho DW.
    Supplementation of vitamin E, vitamin C, and zinc attenuates
    oxidative stress in burned children: a randomized, double-
    blind, placebo-controlled pilot study (2009). *J Burn Care Res.*
    Sep-Oct;30(5):859-66
12. Deloche C, Bastien P, Chadoutaud S, Galan P, Bertrais S,
    Hercberg S, de Lacharrière O. Low iron stores: a risk factor
    for excessive hair loss in non-menopausal women (2007). *Eur J
    Dermatol.* Nov-Dec;17(6):507-12
13. Battaglia Richi E, Baumer B, Conrad B, Darioli R, Schmid A,
    Keller U. Health Risks Associated with Meat Consumption:
    A Review of Epidemiological Studies (2015). *Int J Vitam Nutr
    Res.* 2;85(1-2):70-8
14. Fusano M, Galimberti MG, Bencini M, Fusano I, Bencini PL.
    Comparison of microfocused ultrasound with visualization
    for skin laxity among vegan and omnivore patients (2021). *J
    Cosmet Dermatol.* Sep;20(9):2769-2774

3 THE GUT–SKIN CONNECTION

1. Valdes AM, Walter J, Segal E, Spector TD. Role of the gut
   microbiota in nutrition and health. *BMJ.* 2018 Jun 13;36.
2. Salem I, Ramser A, Isham N, Ghannoum MA. The Gut
   Microbiome as a Major Regulator of the Gut-Skin Axis (2018).
   Front Microbiol. Jul 10;9:1459
3. Goodarzi A, Mozafarpoor S, Bodaghabadi M, Mohamadi
   M. The potential of probiotics for treating acne vulgaris: A
   review of literature on acne and microbiota(2020). *Dermatol
   Ther.* May;33(3)
4. Ragonnaud E, Biragyn A. Gut microbiota as the key controllers
   of "healthy" aging of elderly people (2021). *Immun Ageing.*
   Jan 5;18(1):2
5. Parodi A, Paolino S, Greco A, Drago F, Mansi C, Rebora A,
   Parodi A, Savarino V. Small intestinal bacterial overgrowth
   in rosacea: clinical effectiveness of its eradication (2008). *Clin
   Gastroenterol Hepatol.* Jul;6(7):759-64
6. Agnoletti AF, DE Col E, Parodi A, Schiavetti I, Savarino V,
   Rebora A, Paolino S, Cozzani E, Drago F. Etiopathogenesis of

rosacea: a prospective study with a three-year follow-up (2017). *G Ital Dermatol Venereol.* Oct;152(5):418-423

7. Codoñer FM, Ramírez-Bosca A, Climent E, Carrión-Gutierrez M, Guerrero M, Pérez-Orquín JM, Horga de la Parte J, Genovés S, Ramón D, Navarro-López V, Chenoll E. Gut microbial composition in patients with psoriasis (2018). *Sci Rep.* Feb 28;8(1):3812

8. Zeng L, Yu G, Wu Y, Hao W, Chen H. The Effectiveness and Safety of Probiotic Supplements for Psoriasis: A Systematic Review and Meta-Analysis of Randomized Controlled Trials and Preclinical Trials (2021). *J Immunol Res.* Dec 13;2021:7552546

9. Fiocchi A, Pawankar R, Cuello-Garcia C, Ahn K, Al-Hammadi S, Agarwal A, Beyer K, Burks W, Canonica GW, Ebisawa M, Gandhi S, Kamenwa R, Lee BW, Li H, Prescott S, Riva JJ, Rosenwasser L, Sampson H, Spigler M, Terracciano L, Vereda-Ortiz A, Waserman S, Yepes-Nuñez JJ, Brożek JL, Schünemann HJ. World Allergy Organization-McMaster University Guidelines for Allergic Disease Prevention (GLAD-P): Probiotics (2015). *World Allergy Organ J.* Jan 27;8(1):.

10. McDonald D, Hyde E, Debelius JW, Morton JT, Gonzalez A, Ackermann G, Aksenov AA, Behsaz B, Brennan C, Chen Y et al., American Gut: an Open Platform for Citizen Science Microbiome Research (2018). *mSystems.* May 15;3(3)

11. Wastyk HC, Fragiadakis GK, Perelman D, Dahan D, Merrill BD, Yu FB, Topf M, Gonzalez CG, Van Treuren W, Han S, Robinson JL, Elias JE, Sonnenburg ED, Gardner CD, Sonnenburg JL. Gut-microbiota-targeted diets modulate human immune status (2021). *Cell.* Aug 5;184(16):4137-4153.e14

12. Forslund SK. Fasting intervention and its clinical effects on the human host and microbiome (2023). *J Intern Med.* Feb;293(2):166-183

4 THE SKINFOOD APPROACH

1. Keys A, Menotti A, Aravanis C, Blackburn H, Djordevic BS, Buzina R, Dontas AS, Fidanza F, Karvonen MJ, Kimura N, et al. The seven countries study: 2,289 deaths in 15 years (1984). *Prev Med.* Mar;13(2):141-54

2. Mahamat-Saleh Y, Cervenka I, Al Rahmoun M, Savoye I, Mancini FR, Trichopoulou A, Boutron-Ruault MC, Kvaskoff M. Mediterranean dietary pattern and skin cancer risk: A prospective cohort study in French women (2019). *Am J Clin Nutr.* Oct 1;110(4):993-1002

3. Phan C, Touvier M, Kesse-Guyot E, Adjibade M, Hercberg S, Wolkenstein P, Chosidow O, Ezzedine K, Sbidian E. Association Between Mediterranean Anti-inflammatory Dietary Profile and Severity of Psoriasis: Results From the NutriNet-Santé Cohort (2018). *JAMA Dermatol.* Sep 1;154(9):1017-1024

4. Bertolani M, Rodighiero E, Saleri R, Pedrazzi G, Bertoli S, Leone A, Feliciani C, Lotti T, Satolli F. The influence of Mediterranean diet in acne pathogenesis and the correlation with insulin-like growth factor-1 serum levels: Implications and results (2021). *Dermatol Reports.* Dec 17;14(1):9143

5. Hewlings SJ, Kalman DS. Curcumin: A Review of Its Effects on Human Health (2017). *Foods.* Oct 22;6(10):92

6. Maleki, V, Faghfouri, AH, Tabrizi, FPF *et al.* Mechanistic and therapeutic insight into the effects of cinnamon in polycystic ovary syndrome: a systematic review(2021). *J Ovarian Res.* 14, 130

7. de Cabo R, Mattson MP. Effects of Intermittent Fasting on Health, Aging, and Disease (2019). *N Engl J Med.* Dec 26;381(26):2541-2551

8. Wolf R, Wolf D, Rudikoff D, Parish LC. Nutrition and water: drinking eight glasses of water a day ensures proper skin hydration – myth or reality? (2010). *Clin Dermatol.* Jul-Aug;28(4):380-3

5 OPTIMISING NUTRITION FOR SPECIFIC SKIN CONCERNS

1. Nguyen QG, Markus R, Katta R. Diet and acne: an exploratory survey study of patient beliefs (2016). *Dermatol Pract Concept.* Apr 30;6(2):21-7

2. Berry, S.E., Valdes, A.M., Drew, D.A. et al. Human postprandial responses to food and potential for precision nutrition. *Nat Med* 26, 964–973 (2020)

3. Meixiong J, Ricco C, Vasavda C, Ho BK. Diet and acne: A systematic review (2022). *JAAD Int.* Mar 29;7:95-112

4. Penso L, Touvier M, Deschasaux M, Szabo de Edelenyi F, Hercberg S, Ezzedine K, Sbidian E. Association Between Adult Acne and Dietary Behaviors: Findings From the NutriNet-Santé Prospective Cohort Study (2020). *JAMA Dermatol.* Aug 1;156(8):854-862.

5. Meixiong J, Ricco C, Vasavda C, Ho BK. Diet and acne: A systematic review(2022). *JAAD Int.* Mar 29;7:95-112

6. Rouhani P, Berman B, *et al.* 'Poster 706: Acne improves with a popular, low glycemic diet from South Beach(2009)'. *J Am Acad Dermatol.*;60(3, suppl 1)

7. Aghasi M, Golzarand M, Shab-Bidar S, Aminianfar A, Omidian M, Taheri F. Dairy intake and acne development: A meta-analysis of observational studies (2019). *Clin Nutr.* Jun;38(3):1067-1075

8. Noordam R, Gunn DA, Tomlin CC, Maier AB, Mooijaart SP, Slagboom PE, Westendorp RG, de Craen AJ, van Heemst D; Leiden Longevity Study Group. High serum glucose levels are associated with a higher perceived age(2013). *Age* (Dordr). Feb;35(1):189-95

9. Purba MB, Kouris-Blazos A, Wattanapenpaiboon N, Lukito W, Rothenberg EM, Steen BC, Wahlqvist ML. Skin wrinkling: can food make a difference? (2001) *J Am Coll Nutr.* Feb;20(1):71-80

10. Cosgrove MC, Franco OH, Granger SP, Murray PG, Mayes AE. Dietary nutrient intakes and skin-aging appearance among middle-aged American women (2007). *Am J Clin Nutr.* Oct;86(4):1225-31

11. Hughes MCB, Williams GM, Pageon H, Fourtanier A, Green AC. Dietary Antioxidant Capacity and Skin Photoaging: A 15-Year Longitudinal Study(2021). *J Invest Dermatol.* Apr;141(4S):1111-1118

12. Nagata C, Nakamura K, Wada K, Oba S, Hayashi M, Takeda N, Yasuda K. Association of dietary fat, vegetables and antioxidant micronutrients with skin ageing in Japanese women(2010). *Br J Nutr.* May;103(10):1493-8.

13. de Miranda RB, Weimer P, Rossi RC. Effects of hydrolyzed collagen supplementation on skin aging: a systematic review and meta-analysis (2021). *Int J Dermatol.* Dec;60(12):1449-1461

14. Goodman GD, Kaufman J, Day D, Weiss R, Kawata AK, Garcia JK, Santangelo S, Gallagher CJ. Impact of Smoking and Alcohol Use on Facial Aging in Women: Results of a Large Multinational, Multiracial, Cross-sectional Survey(2019). *J Clin Aesthet Dermatol.* Aug;12(8):28-39

15. Li S, Cho E, Drucker AM, Qureshi AA, Li WQ. Alcohol intake and risk of rosacea in US women(2017). J Am *Acad Dermatol.* Jun;76(6):1061-106

16. Zanesco S, Hall W, Gibson R, Griffiths C, Maruthappu T. Approaches to nutrition intervention in plaque psoriasis, a multi-system inflammatory disease-The Diet and Psoriasis Project (DIEPP)(2022). *Nutr Bull.* Dec;47(4):524-537

17. Mahil SK, McSweeney SM, Kloczko E, McGowan B, Barker JN, Smith CH. Does weight loss reduce the severity and incidence of psoriasis or psoriatic arthritis? A Critically Appraised Topic(2019). Br J Dermatol.Nov;181(5):946-953.

18. Afifi L, Danesh MJ, Lee KM, Beroukhim K, Farahnik B, Ahn RS, Yan D, Singh RK, Nakamura M, Koo J, Liao W. Dietary Behaviors in Psoriasis: Patient-Reported Outcomes from a U.S. National Survey (2017). *Dermatol Ther* (Heidelb). Jun;7(2):227-242

19. Michaëlsson G, Gerdén B, Hagforsen E, Nilsson B, Pihl-Lundin I, Kraaz W, Hjelmquist G, Lööf L. Psoriasis patients with antibodies to gliadin can be improved by a gluten-free diet(2000). *Br J Dermatol.* Jan;142(1):44-51

20. Zhong L, Luo N, Zhong X, Xu T, Hao P. The immunoregulatory effects of natural products on psoriasis via its action on Th17 cells versus regulatory T cells balance (2022). *Int Immunopharmacol.* Sep;110:109032

6 ECZEMA, FOOD ALLERGIES AND INTOLERANCES

1. Du Toit G, Roberts G, Sayre PH, Bahnson HT, Radulovic S, Santos AF, Brough HA, Phippard D, Basting M, Feeney M, Turcanu V, Sever ML, Gomez Lorenzo M, Plaut M, Lack G; LEAP Study Team. Randomized trial of peanut consumption in infants at risk for peanut allergy(2015). *N Engl J Med.* Feb 26;372(9):803-13

7 NURTURING OUR MIND AND OUR SKIN

1. Poli F, Dreno B, Verschoore M. An epidemiological study of acne in female adults: results of a survey conducted in France (2001). *J Eur Acad Dermatol Venereol.* Nov;15(6):541-5

2. Lin J, Epel E. Stress and telomere shortening: Insights from cellular mechanisms (2022). *Ageing Res Rev.* Jan;73:101507

3. Wang Z, Xie H, Gong Y, Ouyang Y, Deng F, Tang Y, Li J. Relationship between rosacea and sleep(2020). *J Dermatol.* Jun;47(6):592-600

4. Aberg KM, Radek KA, Choi EH, Kim DK, Demerjian M, Hupe M, Kerbleski J, Gallo RL, Ganz T, Mauro T, Feingold KR, Elias PM. Psychological stress downregulates epidermal antimicrobial peptide expression and increases severity of cutaneous infections in mice (2007). *J Clin Invest.* Nov;117(11):3339-49

5. Garg A, Chren MM, Sands LP, Matsui MS, Marenus KD, Feingold KR, Elias PM. Psychological stress perturbs epidermal permeability barrier homeostasis: implications for the pathogenesis of stress-associated skin disorders (2001). *Arch Dermatol.* Jan;137(1):53-9

6. Kabat-Zinn J, Wheeler E, Light T, Skillings A, Scharf MJ, Cropley TG, Hosmer D, Bernhard JD. Influence of a mindfulness meditation-based stress reduction intervention on rates of skin clearing in patients with moderate to severe psoriasis undergoing phototherapy (UVB) and photochemotherapy (PUVA) (1998). *Psychosom Med.* Sep-Oct;60(5):625-32

7. Schutte NS, Malouff JM, Keng SL. Meditation and telomere length: a meta-analysis (2020). *Psychol Health.* Aug;35(8):901-915

8. Axelsson J, Sundelin T, Ingre M, Van Someren EJ, Olsson A, Lekander M. Beauty sleep: experimental study on the perceived health and attractiveness of sleep deprived people(2010). *BMJ.* Dec 14;341

9. Cheah KL, Norhayati MN, Husniati Yaacob L, Abdul Rahman R. Effect of Ashwagandha (Withania somnifera) extract on sleep: A systematic review and meta-analysis(2021). *PLoS One.* Sep 24;16(9)

10. Jacka FN, O'Neil A, Opie R, Itsiopoulos C, Cotton S, Mohebbi M, Castle D, Dash S, Mihalopoulos C, Chatterton ML, Brazionis L, Dean OM, Hodge AM, Berk M. A randomised controlled trial of dietary improvement for adults with major depression (the 'SMILES' trial)(2017). *BMC Med.* Jan 30;15(1):23.

Index

Page numbers in *italic* refer to diagrams